Healthy and Quick
& Everything Fit

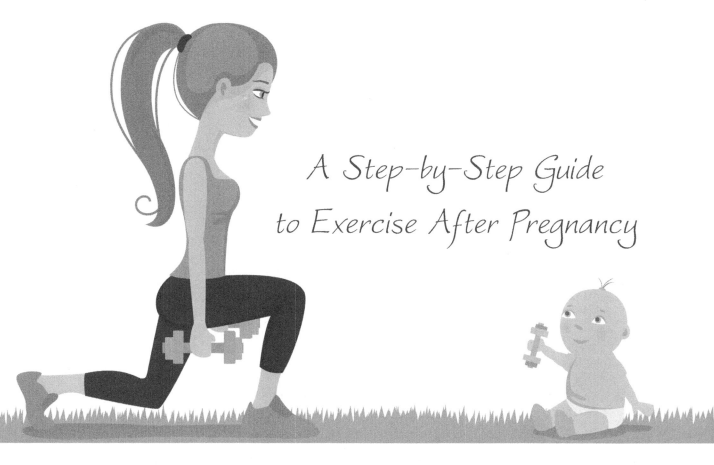

*A Step-by-Step Guide
to Exercise After Pregnancy*

Christine A. Iverson, PT, DPT, OCS
Physical Therapist

Transformation Media Books
Bloomington, Indiana

Published by Transformation Media Books, USA

Transformation Media Books

www.TransformationMediaBooks.com
info@TransformationMediaBooks.com

An imprint of Pen & Publish, Inc.
www.PenandPublish.com
Bloomington, Indiana
(314) 827-6567

Print ISBN: **978-1-941799-25-3**
eBook ISBN: **978-1-941799-26-0**

Cover Illustration: Natalia Lavrinenko

Medical Illustrations:
Delilah Cohn, MFA, CMI, FAMI
Principal | Board Certified Medical Illustrator
The Medical Illustration Studio

Foreword

When Christine brought up the concept for this book, it was one of those moments where I suddenly realized how large a gap existed, and how badly it was needed. In my own practice as a maternal fetal medicine physician, I spend most of my time focusing on getting the mother through pregnancy. But after my own wife was on bedrest for three pregnancies, I realized that I had little to no advice to offer on recovering afterward.

Left without clear evidence or guidance, women have had to try and figure out what works without the tools and understanding they need for success. What this book does is start with the normal changes that happen in pregnancy and then address how to manage them in a clear and systematic way. It also recognizes the clear link between the health of the mother and the health of the baby.

This program is the result of passion and determination. Writing and creating something with this depth and focus is nothing short of amazing. Christine not only believes in this program, but has lived it and I am thankful that she is sharing it so that other women can benefit.

This is a book that is desperately needed and incredibly valuable and I have already started telling my patients about the approach it takes. If knowledge is power, this program is lightning!

Col. Shad Deering, MD
Professor and Chair, Department of Obstetrics and Gynecology, USUHS
Author of *A Practical Manual to Labor and Delivery for Medical Students and Residents*

DISCLAIMER

In no way are this book, the exercises in the photographs, or the accompanying videos meant to replace, counter, or conflict with your physician or your own physical therapist's advice. Before you begin any exercise program, you must consult with a medical health professional, and that is particularly important after giving birth. It is absolutely essential that before beginning this program or any exercise program you consult with your physician about the specific content of the program, including the exercise progression. Every pregnancy and every woman is different, and only your doctor knows your situation. If you have questions about your post-pregnancy health, please consult with your physician, physical therapist, or lactation consultant, as appropriate. Risk for injury is inherent with any exercise program. The exercises in this book are offered with no guarantees on the part of the publisher or the author, and the author and publisher specifically disclaim any and all liability arising directly or indirectly from the use or application of any information contained in this book.

ACKNOWLEDGMENTS

I hope this book is a gift to you and your children as you get back to the movement, sport, or competition that you're passionate about. Writing this book during the first two years of my son's life was a challenge, and I would never have been able to finish this book without the gifts of wisdom, encouragement, and inspiration that my husband, my mother, my sister, my children, and my many professional mentors gave me throughout this endeavor.

My amazing pediatrician, Cate Mason, MD, my wonderful lactation consultant, Ms. Robin Clark, RNC, IBCLC, and my dear friend and longtime mentor, Lisa Hines, PT, DPT, OCS, were my trusted sounding boards and content editors. I sincerely appreciate all of the time and help they gave to me along the way. Even more, I appreciate the passion each one brings to her profession; it is truly an inspiration.

Shad Deering, MD, has encouraged me since this book was simply a question. As an incredibly busy, high-risk obstetrician and Chair of the Department of Obstetrics and Gynecology at Uniformed Services University, he always made time to answer my questions and provide direction. I am incredibly grateful to have such a brilliant professional ally.

My wonderfully patient and talented publisher, Jennifer Geist, has been an absolute joy to work with. Her expertise, knowledge, skill, and encouragement made this book a reality, and for that I am truly grateful.

I couldn't have started, let alone completed, this project without my husband's unwavering support and encouragement. My son did not sleep through the night until he was 19 months old, and I was often up against pure exhaustion while working on this book. Many times I thought about just giving up, but my husband was always there to encourage me, reminding me that he believed in me and telling me that I needed to finish this book because of the potential to help so many fellow moms and their babies. That's what has kept me going.

My own mom and sister inspire me every day. My big sister, who is six years ahead of me on the journey of motherhood with two beautiful daughters, amazed me with her post-pregnancy marathons and commitment to exercise. She has always been there for me, answering motherhood questions in the middle of the night and cheering me on when I have needed it the most.

My mom has been a constant role model and best friend, and as a mother of three and 64-year-old grandmother, she still competes in tennis tournaments across the country. She runs, bikes, and hikes for the love of movement, and that passion to move is something she has passed down to all of her children and grandchildren—a trend I hope to pass to my grandchildren too. She has encouraged me and mentored me as the ultimate athletic mama throughout this whole process, always providing honest and sound advice no matter the time of day or night.

I can't leave out a special thanks to my very own personal trainer, who stuck with me as a running partner from the very first stroller run. Recovering from my pregnancy with my son, David, was the inspiration for this book, and he inspired me every step of the way, literally and figuratively. In the early days he would cry if I wasn't running fast enough. Now that he can tell me what's on his mind, he tells me, "Run faster, Mama!" Way sooner than I can even imagine, he'll be running right next to me.

Very last, but certainly not least, I must thank my littlest contributor, my daughter Jane, who, as I write this acknowledgment, is 37 weeks along in my belly. She has kept me company through the later stages of this project with her little kicks and hiccups, and I hope to always inspire her as much as she already inspires me!

Contents

On the web: www.healthyquickfit.com
Password for exclusive video content available in the **Quick Start Guide** on page **65**

CHAPTER 1
Healing Mom:
An Orthopedic Physical Therapist's Approach

Your post-baby body is triumphant, amazing, stretched, scarred, battle-hardened, and, well . . . jiggly. The changes that your body goes through during the 40 weeks of pregnancy and the rapid, and in some ways traumatic or surgical, changes that happen during delivery are complex and multi-layered. Classifying you as simply "out of shape" is a mistake. In many ways you may be in relatively good shape. Some of your muscles are stronger and your cardiovascular capabilities may be better than before you were pregnant. You are a different shape, yes, than your pre-pregnancy self. If you were on bed rest or unable to exercise during part or all of your pregnancy, you may indeed be out of shape, but your post-pregnancy status actually closely matches that of an athlete recovering from an injury.

I'm writing this book because helping an athlete recover from an injury is what I do best. I'm an orthopedic physical therapist, and I specialize in helping people reach their goals after being sidelined by an injury or surgery. I am also an athlete and a mom, and as I write these pages, my son is nearly 18 months old. I've been in your shoes, and recently. This is the book I wanted to read when I was recovering from my pregnancy. I wanted a detailed, day-by-day program to follow that addressed my post-pregnancy needs. I needed more than the oodles of crunches and planks that make up the bulk of most programs, and as a physical therapist, I could feel the weakness, the tightness, and the altered movement patterns that were affecting me from head to toe, not just my belly. I started to research for this book when my son was a few months old, and I hope to answer your questions about post-pregnancy exercise and provide you with a program that is rooted in the latest research.

I was an Army Physical Therapist for six years, and I spent two of those years serving as the physical therapist for infantry soldiers, then three years with Special Forces soldiers (Green Berets). I went on one deployment with the 101st Airborne Infantry to Iraq in 2007–8, then two deployments back to Iraq in 2009 and 2010 with 5th Special Forces Group as their physical therapist. I am no stranger to helping people to recover from everything from simple ankle sprains to complex chronic injuries to multi-trauma wounds. I know how to help someone without a lot of fancy equipment to heal and train their body for amazing feats and high-demand functioning. You have a few key things in common with infantry and Special Forces soldiers deployed overseas. Moms don't get weekends and nights off. There are no sick days from being a mom, and the physical demands can get pretty tough. Someone else's life is depending on you. Often, you're operating without a lot of sleep. You don't have a lot of time or equipment to work with, and you're on call day and night. We will work together from the inside out to help you heal, retrain your body, prevent injuries, function as a mom, and just maybe get you in the best shape of your life.

I'm going to take an orthopedic physical therapist's approach to helping you because that's what I love to do, what I do best, and that's what I've done for years. I've been able to help a lot of people over the years fix themselves after an injury and get back to doing the things they love and achieve goals they thought were out of their reach. When patients thank me, it's a great feeling, but even better is watching them recover and get back into action. Sometimes a patient will thank me for fixing them or putting them back together, and I always tell them that they fixed themselves; I just gave them good advice.

That's what I want to do for you: advise you in your journey to whole-body fitness after becoming a mother. This program is designed to be a whole-body, daily workout, and it will be challenging. When you are finished with this program, I want you to be able to pursue any of your fitness goals with a balanced, healed, and fit body. Whether you want to train for a marathon, join a local stroller exercise group, or just be as fit as you can be, you'll be ready. You can also continue to use the exercises from any stage of this program indefinitely as a regular routine. Since you are reading this book already, I know you have an interest in exercise, you would like some direction and guidance, and you likely want exercise to be an important part of your baby's life too.

To advise you, I'm going to take the same approach that I take with my orthopedic patients. The key to providing successful advice is figuring out just what structures were involved with the patient's injury, determining what muscle-action patterns have changed, aiming for the patient's goals, and then working from the inside out to put all of the pieces back together. Of course, as a mom you have some challenges that will make your exercise progression unique. You may be worried about how it will affect breastfeeding. You may have questions about exercise and fatigue, postpartum depression, or low back pain. You probably want to know how to avoid getting injured. You also have much more to gain from exercise now that you're a mom, such as the added, lifelong benefits for you now that you're a mom and even more so for your baby. I will address all of that in the first section of this book. The second section will take you day by day through a program designed to recover from all of the pregnancy and delivery related changes, train for the demands of motherhood, get your athleticism and body back, and prevent injuries common among us moms.

What an Orthopedic Physical Therapist Does

Let me take you through a couple of scenarios to give you an understanding of what an orthopedic physical therapist typically does. If you were to get a knee surgery, I would hustle up to your bedside in the hospital with crutches, an exercise band, and a multi-month detailed program to get you back to where you were before your injury. We would start in the hospital room, hours after your surgery, with some exercises you could do in your bed. Later, after leaving the hospital, you would make appointments to see me at my clinic several times a week, and I would guide you through your multi-month program all the way until you were able to run and jump. I'd be regularly checking your strength, motion, and movement patterns. Over the next few months, we'd work on your agility and your core strength, and I'd double-check your running form on the treadmill to look for symmetry.

Let's say instead you had nagging, low back pain that eventually got you to the point that you either wanted my help to get rid of the pain or the pain was preventing you from doing something you wanted to do. You and I would sit down to discuss it. One of my first questions would be, "What happened?" It might be something that developed slowly over time or one incident, such as a fall, that landed you in this situation. Next we would do a lot of digging through your medical history, your daily life, your patterns, your habits, and the things that made your pain worse or better. We would talk about your goals, any barriers you might face, and even your favorite style of learning. Next we would go through a detailed physical exam, looking into all of the possible causes of your problem. We would look for anything we needed to fix, whether it was structural, such as a weakness or tightness, or a movement pattern that needed tweaking. I would give you exercises to do for homework or set you up for exercises or treatment in the clinic, and then we would meet on a regular basis, carefully rechecking your strength, motion, and movement until you were able to reach your goals.

Why an Orthopedic Physical Therapist Can Help You

I would like to say that I was surprised when no physical therapist came to see me when I had my son or that there was no resistance band, no multi-stage program that would get me back to where I was before I was pregnant. The truth is that I knew there would be no physical therapist because I had never gotten a consult to the mother-baby ward myself as a physical therapist. For some reason, we generally see pregnancy and delivery as a self-resolving situation. The most likely reason for you to see a physical therapist after delivering your baby (unless you have an unrelated injury) is for difficulties with continence (control of your bladder and bowel movements). In that scenario, you will see a physical therapist who specializes in the pelvic floor (the muscles that form a hammock at the base of your pelvis). Otherwise, once you have the baby, everything should return to normal on its own, right?

Not quite. After 40 weeks of biomechanical changes followed by the magnificent metamorphosis (and/or surgery) of delivery, you have adopted changes in your movement patterns to compensate for the structural changes, especially in your core. As your pregnancy progressed, you learned to substitute in order to function. After having your baby, your body continues to use these new movement patterns so that you can do all of the things you need to do as a mom, including hefting around your new baby, your new baby's car seat, getting the heavy stroller in and out of the trunk of the car, and all of the other demanding new tasks. As time goes on and you return to more and more challenging tasks and exercises, those movement patterns become habit and weave their way into your everyday life and even your workouts. You neglect the smaller muscles that changed most during your pregnancy or delivery in favor of the larger muscles just to get the job done. Your movements are not as efficient as they once were, and it feels strange the first time you try to run or do a plank because you're using a substituted pattern with muscles that weren't meant for the job. Months or years later, you may become frustrated because you can't do something that you would like to do, your body doesn't work the way you want it to, or you develop an injury from all of your substitutions. Unfortunately, that's when you might meet me, the orthopedic physical therapist.

Goals

Instead of that scenario, I'd like to meet you right now, mom to mom, and take you through how to recover your body the right way. I want you to be able to do all of the things you want to do, whether it's exercise on your own, get started training for a marathon, or join a local stroller group. Stroller exercise groups are a fantastic way to make mommy friends and get a great workout with a group of fellow moms that keeps you motivated. To perform your best and avoid injuries that could sideline you for months, you need to teach your body how to move again by training your core correctly and by targeting all of the deep, smaller muscles before you start working the larger muscle groups. I want you to go to those stroller groups, I want you to train for that marathon, and I want you to build exercise into your daily routine for a lifetime, and when you do, I want your body to be ready, and I want you to know how to exercise the right way so that you can get the most out of it.

The American Congress of Obstetricians and Gynecologists (ACOG) guidelines[1] for returning to exercise following delivery are frustratingly vague. After I had my baby, I wanted to get back to where I was pre-pregnancy (marathon shape). The challenge seemed insurmountable, but the guidance was underwhelming: resume gradually. There is a lot of space between where you are in the mother-baby ward with your post-pregnancy belly and being in the best shape of your life, and I will help you to fill in the blanks. Let's start with that initial question I'd ask you if you came to me in my clinic: What happened?

CHAPTER 2
Effects of Pregnancy on Your Body

Structural Changes

Structurally, your body goes through an amazing array of changes to accommodate your baby during pregnancy. None of these normal structural changes that occur during pregnancy are damaging your body—they are simply your body's incredible way of changing to grow and support a new life. We're going to use the same kind of sleuthing, however, that I use to figure out the best way to help someone heal from an injury in order to help you recover from your pregnancy: we will study the structural changes and altered movement patterns to help guide our focus for your recovery process. Let's start at the bottom and work our way up.

Your Feet

The bony arch of your foot maintains its curved shape with the help of ligaments, muscles, tendons, and fibrous connective tissue. When you are pregnant, the extra body weight, the way you walk (or waddle) when pregnant, and your body's hormonal changes cause that arch to flatten. A flattened arch is more flexible, and the result is a longer foot and the start of a chain reaction that goes right up to your knees and hips. When your foot is flatter, that changes the angle of your ankle, which changes the angle of your knee, which affects the way your hip works too. The changes in your feet are most notable during and after your first pregnancy, but these changes will occur again with any additional pregnancy. Although your feet will naturally regain some of their pre-pregnancy shape after you have your baby, for most women they

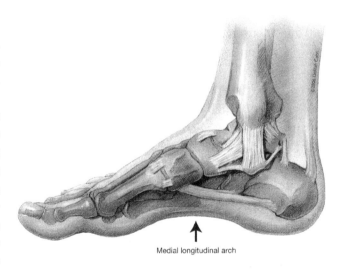

Medial longitudinal arch

Figure 1. Medial foot

will never be quite the same. One in five women will even have a permanent change in shoe size.[2] During this program, we'll work on strengthening the muscles that support your arch to help your feet recover and helping reverse that chain reaction in your lower body that a flattened arch may cause. We'll start with the smaller muscles that are most affected by pregnancy-related changes first, and then we will work in the larger muscles in the more functional movements.

Your Knees

Your knees are actually two joints: one where your thigh bone (femur) meets your shin bone (tibia) and one where your thigh bone meets your kneecap (patella). It's important to the physics of your knees for both joints to be lined up correctly, and your knees can be very sensitive to changes in angle because these changes alter the forces through the bone and affect the way the muscles pull to bend and straighten your knee as you move. When you're pregnant, your knees are affected by the change in angle caused by flattened arches (usually that means they'll angle in a little more), your widening pelvis (causing even more angling in at the knee), and by the change in your center of gravity. The flattened arches can mean more stress on both sides of your knees as well as under your kneecap, and the widening pelvis can change the angle of pull for the thigh muscles that start out at your pelvis and go all the way down to your knees. Even movements as simple as sitting down or standing up can be drastically different with a big belly. When you sit down, for example, with your pregnant belly, you have to reach your bottom way farther back to safely reach the seat and keep your center of gravity over your feet. That translates to a load 1.2 times greater than normal for your thigh muscles every time you sit down, and that begins as early as the second trimester.[3] Over time, that increased stress can add up. During this program, we'll work hard on form as we restore normal movement patterns for basic movements like squatting and lunging, and we'll work to re-strengthen the muscles that were most affected by pregnancy.

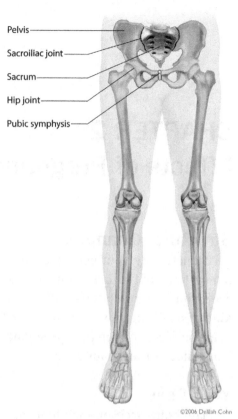

Lower Extremity Alignment

Pelvis —
Sacroiliac joint —
Sacrum —
Hip joint —
Pubic symphysis —

©2006 Delilah Cohn

Figure 2. Lower extremity alignment

Your Pelvis

Your pelvis is actually made up of two large bony structures (each one is made up of three bones fused together) that meet in the front at a joint called your pubic symphysis. Most people are surprised to find out that that bony-feeling structure in the front of your pubic area is actually a joint. It even has a disc and ligaments, and it has to stretch out during pregnancy and delivery to accommodate your baby. Your pelvis joins up in the back with your sacrum, which is the triangle-shaped bone at the bottom of your spine. There is a joint on either side of the sacrum where it meets the pelvis, and those joints are called your sacroiliac joints (SI joints for short). Those joints are covered with ligaments and very strong and tight. Your hip joints are also connected to your pelvis. The socket for each hip joint is on either side of your pelvis. Your pelvis gets some of its stability from the abdominal muscles above it and from the deep hip muscles that surround and go through it as well as the strong ligaments at each joint.

During pregnancy, your abdominal muscles are stretched out and weak, so your pelvis doesn't get a lot of stability from your abdominal muscles.[4,5] At the same time, your pelvis is undergoing lots of changes of its own. The pelvis becomes much more flexible,[6] its degree of tilt changes[6], and overall there's a 10–15% increase in pelvic width.[7] Those changes have a direct effect on the joints of the pelvis, including the pubic symphysis in the front, the hip joints on either side, and the SI joints in the back. The changes to your bony pelvis also have an effect on all of the muscles that attach to the pelvis. That includes muscles of your hips, back, abdomen, and even your shoulders (your lats go all the way from your pelvis to your shoulders).

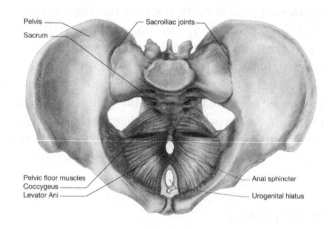

Pelvis —
Sacrum —
Sacroiliac joints —

Pelvic floor muscles
Coccygeus
Levator Ani —

Anal sphincter
Urogenital hiatus

Figure 3. Female pelvis and pelvic floor muscles

Your pelvic floor is at the base of your pelvis and includes some very important muscles that help to make your "core."[8,9] These muscles help control your bladder and bowel movements (keep you from leaking and having accidents),[8-10] assist during sex, support your growing baby during pregnancy, accommodate your baby's route during delivery, and help to stabilize your pelvis.[9] Since the pelvic floor is right at the base of your pelvis, it is also structurally affected by changes in your pelvis's shape and position. The pelvic floor muscles stretch with the weight of your growing baby during pregnancy,[11] and during a vaginal delivery, these muscles stretch even more and in some cases may indeed experience some damage during the delivery process.[12] Even if you had a C-section, your pelvic floor muscles were structurally stretched out during your pregnancy and in some cases even during your labor. Damage to the pelvic floor muscles during delivery is certainly present if there's a grade II or higher tear during delivery or if you undergo an episiotomy (a procedure used to help the baby come out by cutting the tissue between the vagina and anus).[13] During this program, we'll re-stabilize your pelvis by starting each workout with a core drill exercise that incorporates your pelvic floor muscles. We'll work on the deep hip and abdominal muscles that also stabilize your pelvis right away, and as you improve, we'll incorporate more and more challenging and functional movements to incorporate those muscles every step of the way.

Your Hips

Your hip joints are the largest joints in your body. They were built for stability because they connect your legs to your trunk. Your hip joints get their stability from their bony structure (big ball in a pretty deep socket), the strong ligaments and capsule holding the ball in the socket, and the layers of strong muscles that cross the hip joints to help stabilize the joints as you move. The gluteus maximus is also known as your "butt muscle," and it's the best known of all the hip muscles. You also have very important muscles on the outside of your hip that stabilize your hip as you move (especially when you walk and run) as well as rotator muscles to help steer and stabilize your hip and muscles in the front and inside that help generate your movements like walking and running.

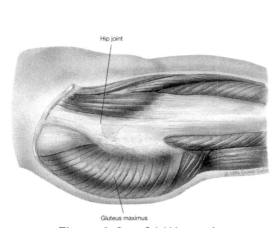

Hip joint

Gluteus maximus

Figure 4. Superficial hip muscles

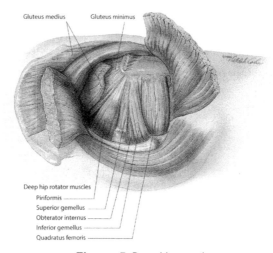

Gluteus medius   Gluteus minimus

Deep hip rotator muscles
Piriformis
Superior gemellus
Obterator internus
Inferior gemellus
Quadratus femoris

Figure 5. Deep hip muscles

As your belly grows, your center of gravity moves forward,[6] and that changes the way you walk and move, which means your hip muscles have to alter the way they work. The new center of gravity plus the altered tilt, width, and stability of the pelvis affect all of your different hip muscles. During pregnancy, your gluteus maximus muscles are operating at a slightly different angle, and there's an increased demand on the muscles on the outside of your hip (gluteus minimus and medius) as your patterns of movement change to accommodate your growing belly.[14] In other words, because of the way you waddle while you walk during pregnancy, you have to use your outer hip muscles more and your butt muscles less to walk. If these outer hip muscles are not strong enough for the new demands, that can eventually lead to low back pain by forcing your body mechanics into unhealthy substitution patterns in order to function.[14] Sometimes these substitution patterns last after you have your baby because you're still carrying a load everywhere you go; you're just carrying it in your arms instead of your belly. To counter these substitution patterns, in this program we will focus on re-training your deep hip muscles first, along their optimal lines of pull, before we do exercises involving multiple hip muscles or in a weight bearing position. Once we bring in the larger muscle groups and complex movements, the smaller muscles will be strong enough to participate correctly in the movement.

Your Belly

Four main muscles make up your abdominal musculature. The most visible is your rectus abdominis, or the six-pack muscle. That's the muscle we're working when we do straight crunches. Next to and just deep to the rectus abdominis are the obliques. The outer oblique muscle is called the external oblique, and the inner oblique muscle is the internal oblique. Their main job is to bend and rotate the spine. The deepest abdominal muscle is your transversus abdominis, or your TrA. That's the muscle you're working when you do a plank (especially a side plank), but planks are only one way of working the TrA (statically). Your TrA works with your deep back muscles to stabilize and decompress your spine. It wraps around your belly like a corset, and it responds to your subconscious by preparing for movements before you even make them. That muscle is key for your core stability and movement patterns. It works together with your diaphragm, deep back muscles, and pelvic floor to make a precise and powerful team that stabilizes your body in static postures and, more importantly, responds to and prepares for movement.

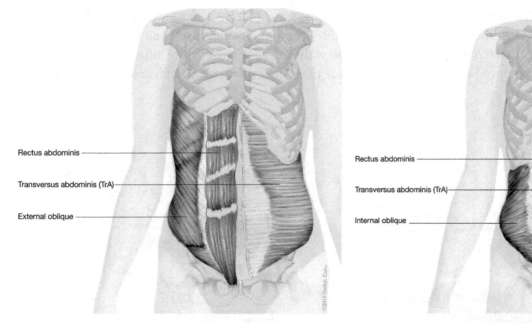

Figure 6. Rectus abdominis, external oblique, and transversus abdominis

Figure 7. Rectus abdominis, internal oblique, and transversus abdominis

As your belly expands to make room for your growing baby, the muscles of your abdomen stretch and weaken.[5,11,15] During pregnancy, the rectus abdominis (six-pack) muscle lengthens, and it also widens at the middle (think of the three cans on either side of the six-pack gradually pulling away from each other in the middle to make room for your baby). This separation is possible because the fibrous tissue between the two sides of the muscle stretches out (don't worry, the tissue doesn't actually tear—it's built to stretch at the center). Separation of that muscle is totally normal during pregnancy, and it usually resolves on its own eight weeks after you have your baby. If the gap between the two sides of the muscle stretches to more than 2.7 centimeters, we describe that situation as a *diastasis recti*.[16] For details about diastasis recti, see Chapter 7.

Your oblique muscles and TrA muscle also blend into fibrous tissue at the center of the belly—they're not meaty muscle tissue all the way around either. Those three muscles and their fibrous center portion also stretch out and weaken during pregnancy to make room for your baby. Since your TrA muscle is involved in stabilizing your trunk to prepare for just about everything you do throughout the day, your body recruits your obliques to try to help stabilize your spine as a substitution pattern when your TrA gets stretched out and weak. Your obliques' main job is to bend and rotate the spine, and they're also stretched out and weak, so they end up doing a fairly poor job when asked to stabilize. During this program we will start working on your deepest layer of abdominal muscles, the TrA first, and work our way out from there. At about six to eight weeks, we'll start working on your other three abdominal muscles. I know you may feel like crunches are the way to get your belly flattened again, but it's important to tighten the inner layer first as we allow the stretched soft tissue to heal in the outer muscles. Exercises that work the TrA will help to bring that stretched soft tissue together, while exercises that work your rectus abdominis and obliques can hinder that healing process by pulling the muscles apart at the center during those first few weeks.

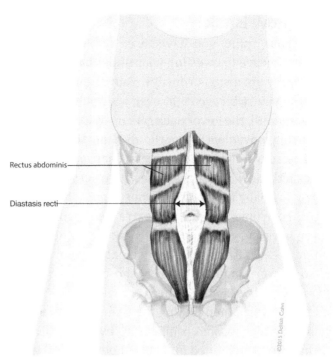

Rectus abdominis

Diastasis recti

©2015 Delsin Cann

Figure 8. Diastasis Recti

Your Low Back

In your spine, you have three natural curves. Your low back is concave (curves in), your upper back is convex (curves out), and your neck is concave. Your S-shaped curve helps to position your rib cage right over your pelvis to keep you centered. Overall, the lower back gets its dynamic stability (stability during movement) from the abdominal and back muscles.

The curve of your lower back changes during pregnancy, but exactly how it changes varies from person to person.[4] With a growing baby in your belly, your center of gravity shifts forward. For some women, the extra belly weight makes their lower back curve deeper,[5,11,15,17] and for others the opposite happens—it flattens out. The weight of your belly pulls your torso forward, and that affects the position of your rib cage over your pelvis. Some women compensate by letting their pelvis tilt forward, then pulling their ribs back to make a deeper S-curve. Other women compensate by tilting their whole pelvis back to keep it lined up under their ribs, and this results in a flattened S-curve.[18] After pregnancy, when the load is still present but in your arms, not your belly, by far the most common tendency is to tilt the pelvis back to keep it positioned under the load in your arms, resulting in a flattened lower back. This could be simply a response to the load in your arms or a combination of the load in your arms and a habit that you picked up during pregnancy to compensate for the load in your belly.[4]

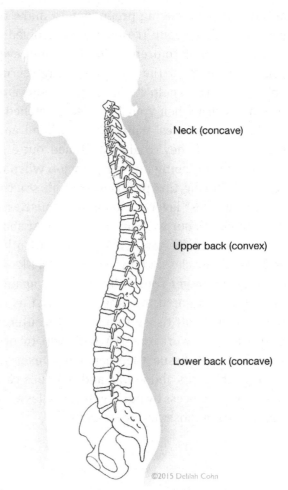

Figure 9. Spinal curvature

Neck (concave)

Upper back (convex)

Lower back (concave)

©2015 Delilah Cohn

Between the weakened and stretched abdominal muscles and the low back muscles pulling at a new angle (whether the curvature is more concave or flattened, it is different), your pregnant and postpartum back just isn't getting the same amount of stability as before you were pregnant. Since you still have to function, you'll pick up substitution patterns that will last until those muscles are strengthened and relearn how to work together post pregnancy.[19] When we strengthen your back during this program, we will be strengthening your core as a whole: working your TrA together with your diaphragm, and pelvic floor. We will also be working on your lower back muscles specifically to re-establish their strength in a healthy, neutral position rather than the position it assumed during your pregnancy (whether your low back was more concave or more flattened).

Your Ribs, Upper Back, and Diaphragm

Your rib cage houses many of your vital organs, including your lungs, and together with your thoracic spine (upper back), your ribs and thoracic spine serve as an attachment point for muscles. One of those muscles is your diaphragm. Its main role is to help you inhale by moving down as it contracts, which opens up space in your lungs, creating negative pressure so you can breathe in. Your diaphragm also has an important role as a part of your core. It works together with your deep abdominal and back muscles and your pelvic floor muscles to create a stable yet dynamic

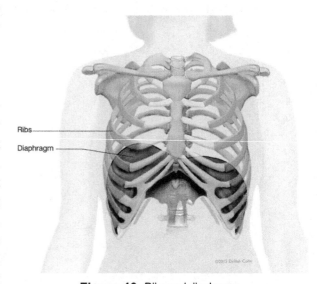

Ribs

Diaphragm

Figure 10. Ribs and diaphragm

core. Your upper back typically has an outward, or convex, curve as part of the S-curve of your spine, which helps to keep your ribs over your pelvis.

During pregnancy, your rib cage expands to create space for your growing baby, increasing in circumference by five to seven centimeters and in diameter from front to back by up to six centimeters.[15,20] Your rib cage flares out as it expands, and your diaphragm shifts up four centimeters above its normal position.[15,20] As the weight of your breasts increases and your ribs change position, your shoulders round forward and your chest muscles become tighter. That causes your upper back to curve out even more.[11] The ability to rotate your upper back side to side is also restricted during pregnancy with all of these adaptive changes.[4]

After you have your baby, your ribs and diaphragm go back to their usual position over time, but for many women, the upper back continues to curve out more and more because of all of the time new moms spend in a hunched-forward position feeding and caring for the baby. From the start we'll be working on restoring the rotation in your upper back, stretching your chest muscles, and strengthening the muscles that pull your shoulders back to help improve your daily movements and counter the hunched posture that affects so many new moms.

Your Head and Neck

The S-curve of your spine continues up to your neck. Since your upper back is convex (curves out), your neck is concave (curves in) so that your head can be right over your shoulders. The muscles deep in your throat (along the front of your spine) and at the base of your skull work together to keep your head and neck in the right position.

When your upper back curves out more, you have to deepen the S-curve at your neck in order to keep your head over your shoulders. That's a lot of work for the tiny muscles at the base of your skull. As those muscles tighten and pull to hold your head up, the deep throat muscles get stretched out and weak. Over time you'll develop what we call "forward head posture" with your ears far forward of your shoulders. This posture can result in neck pain, upper back pain, and headaches. The headaches that are most common from forward head posture are "ram's horn" headaches that start at the base of the skull, go behind the ears, and end over your eyebrows.

In this program, we will start working on stretching these muscles at the base of your skull right away, at the same time that we start work on countering the hunched, upper back posture to nip this problem in the bud.

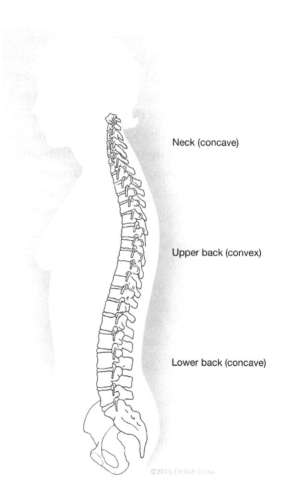

Neck (concave)

Upper back (convex)

Lower back (concave)

©2015 Delilah Cohn

Figure 11. Spinal curvature

The Overall Effects of Pregnancy on Your Body

General Changes

Pregnancy changes your body literally from head to toe in a beautiful, miraculous, and incredible way to give your baby its first home. Average weight gain during pregnancy ranges anywhere from 20 to 41 pounds,[5,17,18,20] or roughly 25 percent of your pre-pregnancy body weight.[15] Your uterus will become 10 times heavier during pregnancy than your pre-pregnancy uterus.[20] Nutritionally, pregnancy requires about an extra 300 kcal per day.[17] Full disclosure, I gained 31 percent of my pre-pregnancy body weight during my first pregnancy. (My second pregnancy is still underway but appears to be headed the same direction.) On average, moms keep about 5 pounds of fat mass after having the baby.[20]

One of the first changes to occur during pregnancy is an increase in heart rate at rest and during a workout. This starts between weeks two and five of your pregnancy[21] and may explain why you started to feel fatigued during your workouts right before you found out you were pregnant. Another early change is an increase in blood volume. By just the sixth week of your pregnancy, your blood volume increases by 30–40 percent. Blood is made up of liquid (plasma) and blood cells. The increase in blood volume during pregnancy is mostly plasma, so some women will experience anemia because the blood cells are diluted.[17,21] Because of the increase in blood volume, your heart is pumping more blood with every beat, and as your pregnancy progresses, you'll be pumping even more blood because you'll have an increase in heart rate in addition to the increase in volume.[17]

Although your diaphragm moves up to accommodate your growing baby during pregnancy, your rib cage expands enough that the net result is an increase in your overall lung capacity.[15,17] Just after having your baby, you are actually poised nicely to exercise because your VO$_2$ max (the rate at which your body takes in oxygen by breathing and distributes it throughout your body—AKA your fuel economy) actually increases. During walking and running, you will have significantly better fuel economy (VO$_2$ max) while pregnant compared to your pre-pregnant self. If you exercise during your pregnancy, the effects are even greater, and if you continue to exercise after having your baby, you can retain that VO$_2$ max improvement.[21]

> **Pregnancy Brain**
>
> While the rest of your body is growing during pregnancy, your brain actually temporarily shrinks, according to a 2002 study out of the UK. The reduction in brain size ranged from 2 to 6.6 percent, but this small amount was statistically considered significant. All of the brains in this study thankfully returned to their normal size six months after delivery. It's not clear yet what causes this change, and, of course, the authors were careful to point out that they could not make any further speculation about what these findings mean[22] (a smart move, lest those of us who experienced "pregnancy brain" jump to conclusions).

During pregnancy, your body increases the production of a hormone called relaxin. Relaxin is a really cool-sounding hormone because it does what it sounds like it ought to: it works together with progesterone to relax the soft tissue throughout your body so that you are able to accommodate and then deliver your baby.[17] Estrogen helps to increase its effects by making your joints more receptive to the relaxin.[23] Relaxin increases to 10 times pre-pregnancy levels during your pregnancy,[18] and though it mostly affects your pelvis, it affects all of your other joints as well.[15,17,18] Relaxin sometimes gets a bad rap as the primary suspect for causing injuries. Logically, it seems like if so much relaxin is affecting the body, wouldn't that make everything unstable and cause injuries? In reality, research hasn't shown relaxin levels to be a major factor in pelvic pain,[6] but having relaxin at such a high level in your body can theoretically increase your risk for injury if a joint is stretched well beyond its normal range.[24] Since relaxin is still present in your system at high levels for the first six–eight weeks after delivery,[5] stretching will only be a minor focus for this program during those first few weeks.

CHAPTER 3
Effects of Pregnancy on the Way You Move

At this point I'd like to start changing your view of your core. Most women know that their core is more than just their six-pack abdominal muscles, that there's something deeper in there that helps to connect and stabilize their whole body, and that the plank is a really good exercise for working your core. Because we're usually pretty interested in getting a flat belly (who isn't?), especially after pregnancy, we tend to think mostly about the abdominal part of our core. Let me introduce you to the other three parts of your core so that you can start thinking of your core less as a deep, stiff rectangle behind your belly and more like a sphere that moves when you move. Structurally and functionally, every part of your core is affected during pregnancy. Your pelvic floor sits at the base of the core, the diaphragm is at the top, your deep back muscles are in the back, and your deep abdominal muscles are in the front. They work together in a specific order to stabilize your body before every movement. These muscles fire in a particular sequence—a rapid progression of muscles turning on *and* off in order to allow for movement—but provide a stable center at just the right moment, so the stability you get from your whole core team of muscles working together is *dynamic*. Plank exercises are great for strengthening some of your core muscles statically, but you also need to train your core dynamically to teach the core muscles to work together in the right way so that they can operate when you exercise and function throughout the day. Holding your TrA tight strengthens that particular muscle, but that type of training alone ignores the rest of your core (remember, your core is a sphere, not a board), and it does not teach your core to function well as a team. Too much static training without dynamic training can actually lead to lots of problems over time.

Movement Patterns: Motor Control

In 1992, the United States was finally allowed to have NBA players participate in the Olympics. The first, second, and third "Dream Teams" won gold medals in 1992, 1996, and 2000. The USA Dream Team is made up of the best basketball players in the country (many agree they are the best individual players in the world) who come together from a variety of NBA teams to play together for Team USA. In 2004, the United States lost to Puerto Rico, Lithuania (the first round), and Argentina. Here's what Coach Larry Brown had to say: "I'm humiliated, not for the loss—I can always deal with wins and losses—but I'm disappointed because I had a job to do as a coach, to get us to understand how we're supposed to play as a team and act as a team, and I don't think we did that." So there you have it. You can have the best individual players in the world, but if they can't work together as a team, they will fail.

What does the 2004 Dream Team have in common with post-pregnancy rehab and fitness? Teamwork. Movement patterns. Motor control. Motor control is your body's ability to use the correct muscle and movement patterns in order to function. We will refer to motor control as movement patterns to be consistent. Your muscles have to work together as a team to perform the most fundamental tasks for daily functions. Most of the time you don't even know it's happening because your body is able to do it subconsciously. When a team member is injured, the rest of the team will pick up the slack and work harder and in new ways in order to accomplish a task.

When a completely healthy person picks up a gallon of milk, a cascade of events happens before she even reaches for the milk. Her diaphragm gets set (regardless of whether she's breathing in or out at that very moment, her diaphragm performs a preparatory contraction).[25] Next, her pelvic floor contracts, and then immediately afterwards her transversus abdominis (deepest abdominal muscle) and multifidus (deepest stabilizing back muscle) fire to stabilize her core. Finally, she moves her arm. Immediately afterwards, the outer abdominal and back muscles fire in response to the weight shift caused by the arm movement. The ability of the diaphragm to fire before you move your limbs occurs even with simple elbow movements.[25]

Let's take a brief look at each of these four core team players: your diaphragm, your pelvic floor, your transversus abdominis (TrA), and your multifidus. We'll look at what each muscle does individually and then examine how they work together as a team with another important piece of the puzzle—the pressure in your abdomen that is getting pushed around during your muscle contractions.

Diaphragm

Your diaphragm has two jobs. It helps you to breathe in and adds to the stability of your pelvis and spine. Your diaphragm is a parachute-shaped muscle that separates your abdominal cavity from your chest cavity. It is attached to your lower six ribs and your upper three lumbar vertebrae. To breathe in, your diaphragm contracts and moves down, creating more space above the diaphragm in your chest so that your lungs can fill with air. When it does that, it increases the pressure down below in your abdomen, and that pressure in your abdomen helps to stabilize and unload the spine.[25]

Functionally, the diaphragm sets up your core team for action like a springboard. When you breathe in, the diaphragm moves down, increasing the pressure in your abdomen.[25] When you breathe out, the pressure in the abdomen decreases, making it easier to perform a pelvic floor and abdominal muscle contraction and tighten your core as you prepare to move your arms or legs.[9,25] When you breathe in, you're getting stability from the core team through an increase in abdominal pressure (loaded springboard). When you breathe out, the pressure in your abdomen decreases (released springboard), but at that very moment, the drop in pressure allows the pelvic floor and abdominal muscles to kick in and provide muscular stability.

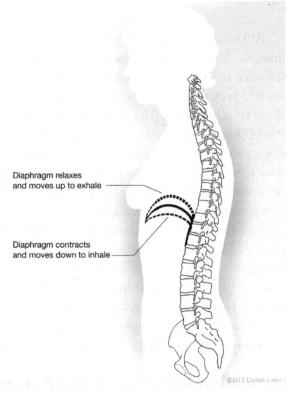

Diaphragm relaxes and moves up to exhale

Diaphragm contracts and moves down to inhale

©2015 Delilah Cohn

Figure 12. Diaphragm in action

Pelvic Floor

Your pelvic floor also performs two main functions: maintaining control of urine and bowel function and stabilizing the pelvis.[8] These muscles also have important roles during sex, pregnancy, and delivery. The pelvic floor is made up of a group of muscles that forms a hammock-shaped structure at the base of your pelvis. The main pelvic floor muscles are known as the levator ani complex: a U-shaped sling that goes around your urethra, vagina, and rectum.[12] They're particularly active when you cough or sneeze, lift heavy objects, or move your arms and legs.[8,9]

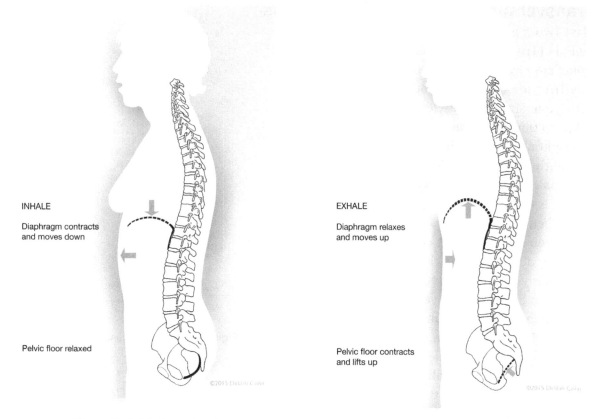

INHALE

Diaphragm contracts
and moves down

Pelvic floor relaxed

©2015 Dehlin Conn

EXHALE

Diaphragm relaxes
and moves up

Pelvic floor contracts
and lifts up

©2015 Dehlin Conn

Figure 13. Pelvic floor relaxed   **Figure 14.** Pelvic floor firing

When you cough or sneeze, your abdominal muscles contract swiftly and hard, increasing the pressure in your abdomen.[9] To prevent leaks or accidents from the increase in pressure, your pelvic floor is able to contract just before that cough or sneeze to pull upwards on the bladder neck and close off your exits.[10] Before you lift heavy objects or move your arms and legs, you're going to contract your abdomen to create a stable base for your limbs.[8] Just like before the cough or sneeze, your pelvic floor muscles fire just ahead of the abdominal contraction to prevent leaks or accidents from the increased pressure and add stability to the pelvis to help create a stable base.[8,9]

The Pelvic Floor: Always On

Research of the pelvic floor muscles has shown that they are always "on," but they have bursts of increased activity before trunk or limb movements to help with both continence and stability.[9,26] Research has also given us some insight about the pelvic floor's usual patterns during quiet breathing. It's "on" whether we're breathing in and breathing out, but a little more "on" when we're breathing out.[9] When we're breathing out, the abdominal pressure is lower, and that makes it easier for the pelvic floor to contract.

23

Your Transversus Abdominis and Multifidus

The last two members of our team, our transversus abdominis (TrA) and multifidus, work together to form a complete circuit around your abdomen, like a corset. The TrA goes all the way around your abdomen, underneath your six-pack muscle and your obliques, and attaches to fibrous tissue in your back. Your multifidus sits right along your vertebrae in the back. The TrA fires slightly earlier than the multifidus, but they fire together as a team.[25] The main function for both of those muscles is to stabilize your spine, and when they contract together, they decompress your spine.

Any time you move, the TrA contracts before you move your other abdominal muscles or your limbs. One thing that makes your TrA so special is that it has the same contraction before you move your limbs regardless of the direction of limb movement. All of your other abdominal muscles fire according to the direction of limb movement. The primary role of the TrA is simply to prepare for any movement at all.[27] Its main job is to stabilize.

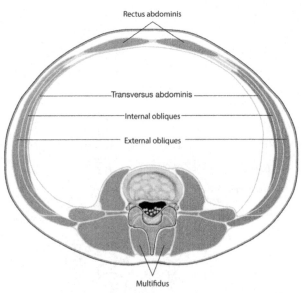

Figure 15. Abdominal muscles cross-section

The TrA has gotten a lot of attention in the past several years as the key figure for core strength, which is great because the TrA is truly an important muscle for core stability and preventing and treating low back pain. The downside to the TrA craze, however, is that we sometimes forget that the TrA is just one member of the team. With all the hype, the TrA gets lots of practice while the rest of our core team gets neglected. If we're just focusing on planks and static exercises alone to strengthen our core, we're doing two things wrong: we're working on static postures rather than the dynamic movements that more closely resemble daily functioning and athletic movements, and we're only strengthening one side of the sphere that makes up our core.

Working Together as a Team

To do "core" work 10 or 15 years ago meant to do lots and lots of crunches. Thankfully the TrA has become a little famous (most people couldn't tell you its name, but nowadays it's more well known that there's a deeper muscle there than your six-pack). Planks are super popular because they are great for working the TrA. Here's the problem: we can't function well if we just have a really strong TrA that's always firing. So while planks are an important part of our program, there's much more to the equation. When we fire our TrA, it co-contracts with the multifidus to create that corset effect. Tightening a corset around our waist spikes the abdominal pressure, meaning that the pressure heads north and south. Pressure moves north towards our diaphragm and south towards our pelvic floor. Our pelvic floor is closely linked to our TrA (both are getting marching orders from the brain and spinal cord), so just before a TrA contraction, the pelvic floor contracts milliseconds earlier.[28] Likewise, if we contract our pelvic floor muscles to do a Kegel, we will get an involuntary contraction of our TrA and obliques.

If we hold that contraction tight as we continue to move and function, it becomes a challenge to take a deep breath and it puts a lot of stress on our pelvic floor muscles, which can lead to trouble with continence and pelvic stability. To function correctly, the TrA and multifidus must work together with the diaphragm and the pelvic floor as a constantly moving pressure transfer system.

Let's take a look at a full sneeze to get an idea of how the whole team works together. Just before you sneeze, you take a deep, rapid breath. Your diaphragm contracts and moves down to allow air into your lungs and compress your abdomen. That's the "AH" part of your sneeze. That pressure in your abdomen is the loaded springboard. Just as you release the springboard, the pelvic floor contracts to block any leaks or accidents in anticipation of a strong abdominal contraction. When the abdominal contraction happens (the "CHOO" part of the sneeze), the shift in pressure forces the sneeze out by pushing upwards on the chest cavity. The same thing happens, except with far less drama, when you pick up your baby or perform really any function in daily life. The muscle pattern, over and over and over again throughout the day, is diaphragm first, pelvic floor second, TrA and multifidus third, and then the functional movement.[10,26,27]

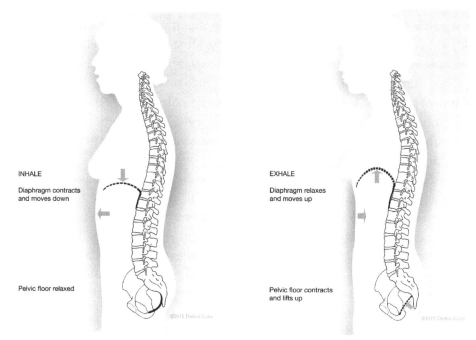

INHALE

Diaphragm contracts
and moves down

Pelvic floor relaxed

EXHALE

Diaphragm relaxes
and moves up

Pelvic floor contracts
and lifts up

Figure 16. "AH" part of sneeze   Figure 17. "CHOO" part of sneeze

Your Post-Pregnancy Core Team

Pregnancy changes the whole way our core team works. During pregnancy, our pelvic floor muscles and TrA stop working together completely.[29] Normally, these two muscles work hand in hand, one causing the other to fire (voluntarily firing either one will cause a contraction in the other).[10,28-30] They are normally so tight-knit, in fact, that firing either one by itself during urination can stop the flow of urine just as well and just as quickly, and that's a job we typically understand as the pelvic floor's main role.[28]

> **A Broken Link**
>
> A study in Brazil checked the core muscle teamwork of 81 women—some who had never been pregnant, some who were pregnant, and some who had recently had babies (they had given birth less than 2 months before the study, either vaginally or via C-section). The pregnant women and new moms had lost the automatic link between the pelvic floor and the TrA that causes one to contract in response to the other firing. Only those who had never been pregnant showed a link between the abdominal muscles and the pelvic floor.[29] As you can imagine, that broken link has a major effect on your core team.

Sometimes a pelvic floor problem shows up as a loss of the ability to control for urine leaks or bowel accidents. People usually aren't very public about their leaks and accidents, but it's more common than you may think. Fifty-eight percent of women who had a vaginal delivery have some form of pelvic floor disorder, and forty-three percent of those who had a cesarean section have some form of pelvic floor disorder (including stress incontinence, overactive bladder, pelvic organ prolapse, or fecal incontinence). Age is a risk factor for developing a pelvic floor disorder after giving birth (moms between the ages of 30 and 44 at the time they gave birth), as is having more children (the risk increases with each one), having an operative vaginal birth (forceps or vacuum assisted birth), and obesity.[12]

Loss of ability to control urine leaks or bowel accidents is an obvious sign that there's a problem with the pelvic floor, but it doesn't necessarily mean that the pelvic floor is weak. You could have a strong pelvic floor after doing lots of Kegel exercises, but if the muscles don't fire in the right order, you won't be able to prevent leaks or accidents. Likewise, just because you don't have leaks or accidents doesn't mean your pelvic floor is working properly. A pelvic floor problem could be so subtle that it only shows up as the root of a troublesome injury or low back pain years after you have your last baby. Most likely, the pelvic floor problem in that case will go unnoticed, and your injury will frustrate you as well as your care providers. It's important to get started now in retraining those muscles the right way to prevent future problems.

If you do have a problem with leaks or accidents or pelvic pain, you need to talk to your doctor about it right away. Don't be embarrassed; your doctor is there to help you, and remember, it's very common. Also, this type of pelvic floor problem often resolves within the first three months after giving birth, but may last a year or longer.[31] Talk to your doctor anyway. Depending on your situation and your doctor's assessment, you may get consulted to a physical therapist who specializes in the pelvic floor. If you have a problem with your pelvic floor, pelvic floor physical therapy can be life-changing for you, and I urge you to please seek help. The exercises we will go through in this book are written for everybody who has had a baby (not intended as therapy to fix problems with leaks or accidents), but they can be a part of your program if you are seeing a pelvic floor physical therapist for leaks and accidents as well. If you are undergoing physical therapy for your pelvic floor problem, please *take this book with you* to your pelvic floor physical therapist and show her the exercises in the book. Have her decide how and when to work them into your program. Whether you have a known pelvic floor problem or not, you should have a physical therapist or your obstetrician check your pelvic floor and/or TrA muscle contraction before you get started with this program to make sure you have the basics right.

Timing is Everything

Here is what we have learned from researching women with the obvious pelvic floor problems that cause leaks and accidents: timing is everything. When continent women (women without a problem with leaks or accidents) move their arms rapidly, their pelvic floor muscle activity increases *before* the arm movement, but when incontinent women do the same thing, their pelvic floor muscles fire *after* the arm movement. Remember, the Dream Team is supposed to work like this: contract diaphragm, contract pelvic floor, contract TrA and multifidus, move limbs. Recent research has revealed three striking findings. First, for most women with incontinence, pelvic floor activity actually *decreases* before limb movement. Second, incontinent women often actually have stronger activity of their pelvic floor muscles than continent women—they just fire the pelvic floor muscles later. Third, incontinent women often fire their abdominal muscles before their pelvic floor muscles.[8] So here's what happened in the incontinent women studied: contract diaphragm, contract abdominal muscles, *decrease* pelvic floor activity (in most), move limb, then contract pelvic floor muscles *really hard* to make up for firing late and to make a last-ditch effort to catch leaks or accidents.

Another study found similar results with continent versus incontinent women during coughing. In this recent study, both groups of women were able to reach about the same level of pelvic floor activity, but the difference again was in the timing. Those with incontinence fired their abdominal muscles before their pelvic floor muscles when coughing, and the continent women fired their abdominal muscles *after* their pelvic floor muscles when coughing.[26] Again, timing is everything.

How to Repair Your Core Team

During our program, we're going to train your transversus abdominis muscle both as a team member and with some isolated TrA work to get the muscle activating and strengthened again. Just getting the muscle to contract and strengthen is important,[32] but we are going to respect the multidimensional complexities of this muscle[10] and train it as a member of a team by consistently focusing on timing, multidirectional movements, and functional drills.

Likewise, when we train your pelvic floor, we're going to take it out of isolation. It's still a good idea to do Kegel exercises throughout the day, but during this workout program your pelvic floor exercises will be incorporated with other exercises. Sometimes women receive advice to relax their abdominal muscles completely to do a correct Kegel exercise, but there's some recent research that suggests that this advice is not only unrealistic, but can be counterproductive.[33] The pelvic floor does not function in isolation, so training it while trying to keep the abdominal muscles completely relaxed can lead to faulty patterns of movement.

Exercises like the "knack," whereby you consciously contract your pelvic floor muscles just before you cough or sneeze, are helpful because they are exercises that focus on timing as well as strength.[8] We will bring the "knack" up a notch and perform a drill called the "piston," designed by a brilliant pelvic floor physical therapist named Julie Weibe from California. Her work inspired and helped to guide my research for this chapter. The idea during the piston exercise is to perform the core team contractions in the correct order as a pre-set for another exercise, like a squat: diaphragm, pelvic floor, TrA and multifidus, then move your trunk or limbs. We are going to incorporate the piston exercise by starting each workout with progressively more functional core drills to prime your core teamwork.

Normal Movement Pattern	Post-Pregnancy Movement Pattern
Decide to pick up object	Decide to pick up object
Diaphragm contracts (whether breathing in or out at the moment)	Diaphragm contracts (whether breathing in or out at the moment)
Pelvic floor fires	Deep abdominal muscle (TrA) and back muscles (multifidi) fire (disorganized pattern)
Deep abdominal muscle (TrA) and back muscles (multifidi) fire	Fire outer abdominal muscles
Fire some outer abdominal muscles to help prep for movement, depending on direction of movement	**Move arm to get object**
Move arm to get object	Fire other abdominal muscles to respond to weight shifting from arm movement
Fire other abdominal muscles to respond to weight shifting from arm movement	**Fire pelvic floor muscles really hard to try to make up for the late timing**

Movement Pattern Changes: Not Just Your Pelvic Floor

Changes in movement patterns happen throughout your body during your pregnancy, not just in your core. Let's look at the way you walk, for example. Because of the change in your weight distribution and the change in your center of gravity, you start to use your muscles in a different way to walk. Pregnant women take shorter and wider steps. To walk with these shorter and wider steps, your body recruits the muscles on the outside of your hips to walk instead your butt muscles. Your butt muscles work to move your leg back when you walk, but with a side-to-side (also known as waddling) gait, you have to use the outer hip muscles more and the butt muscles less. During pregnancy, you also rotate your body at a different latitude to walk. Normally we rotate our trunk with each step during walking, but during pregnancy that rotation comes from the pelvis, and our trunk becomes more rigid.[4] Changes to your walking patterns and muscle recruitment patterns happen in exact proportion to the structural changes in your body. In other words, the more you grow, the more your walking patterns change.[18]

After pregnancy, it is important to relearn even the most basic movement patterns for your non-pregnant body. The angle of pull for the muscles is different and the patterns of movement are different after you've had the baby. To get the muscles to work correctly again, we will need to awaken and strengthen muscles that weren't used as much during pregnancy and reteach all of the muscles affected by your pregnancy how to work together as a team again for even the most basic functions.

Optimal Post-Pregnancy Training

We often make one of two mistakes post-injury. One mistake is going right into functional, large muscle group movements without training the injured or affected muscles first. Let's say, for instance, that you were to go for a run two weeks after having your baby. Could you physically do it? Probably (though I don't know if any obstetrician or physical therapist would advise that). Would it be painful or uncomfortable? Probably. Would you be running at your best? Of course not, because the movement patterns you adopted during your pregnancy were substitution patterns that left out key muscles affected by your pregnancy. You would likely continue that substituted movement pattern indefinitely unless you went back to the basics at some point and retrained the muscles and movement patterns affected by your pregnancy.

The second mistake is training each body part separately, never putting the pieces together or training as a team. That's the 2004 Dream Team mistake, and it's most common with our core muscles. We train our pelvic floor with Kegel exercises, we do planks, we do crunches, we hold our bellies rigid and tight doing lots of different exercises to get that transversus abdominis as strong as we possibly can, but we never train the team together in the right order. We can have a wonderfully strong transversus abdominis, do a killer set of Kegels, and still have trouble with functional movements or even continence because those core team players just can't work together. That is the key mistake the best of us sometimes make in rehab. During this program, we will start with basic movements to activate muscles that were most affected by your pregnancy. At the same time we will start working on basic drills to re-establish your movement pattern timing. As you improve, we will work on strengthening, then add balance and functional movements, all the while continuing progressively more difficult timing drills.

CHAPTER 4
Benefits of Exercise for Mom

Benefits of Exercise for Mom

Just after you've had a baby is the best time of your life to begin or continue exercising for two reasons. First, at this point in your life you actually stand to gain a lot more from exercise than at any other time. Second, it will be more difficult to work exercise into your schedule now than ever before and at any time in the future.[34] Why would a time crunch make it the best time to start or continue exercising? As a mother, you will be orchestrating a precise daily schedule. Time will no longer be linear, but divided into chunks throughout the day. The framework of your daily life changes drastically with the birth of your baby. At first, you will live in repeating three-hour intervals. As your baby grows older, those chunks will become more complex and variable. If you have more than one child, you'll be orchestrating a symphony rather than a duet. As you know, exercise takes time, effort, and discipline. A large enough chunk of time to exercise will be harder to come by now than ever before. If you prioritize it into your schedule now, it will have staying power for you and the rest of your family.

Since you're reading this book, I know you're already sold on exercise. You know that the benefits of exercise include improved strength and cardiovascular fitness, improved functional capabilities, improved physique and decreased risk for obesity, improved joint health, decreased risk for chronic diseases such as cardiovascular disease, diabetes, and some cancers, and a greater chance of living longer. There will be days, however, when you need just a little extra nudge to help you get your workout in. You may be feeling frazzled, sluggish, or maybe even guilty for spending time taking care of yourself. Please don't feel guilty about exercising. Exercise will benefit you and your whole family on a daily basis and in the long-term. I'll fill you in on the benefits of exercise that are specific to mothers to help give you a little extra boost on those tough days.

Right Away: Benefits in the Hospital

The added benefits of exercise for mothers begin right away in the hospital. If you are able to do some light exercise (such as slow walking around the hallways or simple ankle pumps in your bed) while you're still in the hospital, you'll have improved circulation and reduce your risk for swelling and blood clots, and you'll begin the first steps to restore the muscles stressed during your pregnancy and delivery.[34] Before you do any exercise in the hospital (even walking laps in the hallway), discuss your intentions with your obstetrician. Every pregnancy and delivery is different, and it's important for your safety to take the opportunity while you're in the hospital to discuss your exercise plans with your obstetrician—any exercises you plan to do while you're still in the hospital as well as this plan. If you are reading this book before you have your baby, take this book with you as a part of your overnight bag in the hospital and show it to your doctor for approval. If you've already had your baby, discuss this program with your obstetrician or your primary care provider before beginning.

Once you begin a daily exercise program after leaving the hospital, you'll begin to experience some direct and relatively immediate benefits, such as the beginnings of an improved physique,[35] an overall improvement in fitness and cardiovascular health,[24,34,36] improved blood chemistry,[24,34,35] and improved bone density.[37]

Preventing Becoming Overweight and Obesity

For mothers more than anyone else, exercise after pregnancy is an important part of preventing obesity and becoming overweight. Right now, over 71 percent of women in the United States are overweight (BMI over 25 but less than 30), obese (BMI between 30 and 40), or extremely obese (BMI 40 or more).[38] Only 26 percent of American women get the American College of Sports Medicine-recommended 30 minutes of moderate physical activity on most or all days of the week.[21] Moderate physical activity doesn't need to be a spin class or a trail run. Moderate physical activity includes simple activities that may already be a part of your daily life, such as brisk walking or even heavy housework like vacuuming or taking in the groceries, and 74 percent of American women are not getting 30 minutes of that in per day. On average, mothers keep 1–4 pounds of extra weight per child, but about 14 percent of women keep more than 10 pounds of extra weight per child.[39] At one year after giving birth, moms average 1–6 pounds more than their pre-pregnancy weight. At the one year mark, 14 to 20 percent of women are still 10 pounds or more above their pre-pregnancy weight at the one year mark.[40] Overall, the risk of becoming overweight increases by 60 percent and the risk of becoming obese increases by 110 percent after having one baby.[39] Exercise is even more important for mothers because we are at higher risk for becoming overweight or obese.

The good news is that exercise and fitness during that first year of your baby's life are major factors in preventing becoming overweight and obesity down the road. While moms who exercise don't lose more weight than the non-exercisers during the first few months after giving birth[39] (more powerful forces are at work here during the first few months, but more on that later), women who exercise in the first year after giving birth gain less weight during later years than those who did not exercise during that time.[40] So while you may not look much different from your non-exercising friends during the first few months after having your baby, you will reap the benefits for decades later. Your weight at the one-year mark after giving birth is a predictor of weight gain even 15 years later—if you come within about 3–4 pounds of your pre-pregnancy weight by the time your baby turns 1, you are much less likely to be overweight when your baby turns 15.[41]

Exercise and Diet: Dynamic Duo

When you're exercising to improve your body image and to lose weight after having a baby, nutrition is an important factor. Some studies show that exercising after giving birth increases your chances of returning to your pre-pregnancy weight and that in the long term (eight to ten years) you'll gain less weight than moms who don't exercise.[34,35] Other studies show that exercise alone will not help you to lose body weight unless you are also watching what you eat.

Exercise? Diet? Both?

One recent, large-scale review of 14 studies on the topic found that overall, exercise will improve your cardiovascular fitness, but in the first year after you give birth, exercise without a proper diet will not result in significant weight loss. Dieting without exercise will result in weight loss, but you'll be losing lots of lean body mass (you're interested in losing fat mass, not lean mass). The combination of a good diet plus exercise had the best results: these moms lost significant weight without losing lean body mass.[41] If you are interested in improving or altering your diet in conjunction with this program, ask your doctor for a consult to see a dietician. She will be able analyze your diet and provide guidance about a diet that will be good for you and for your baby if you are breastfeeding.

Improved Response to Insulin and Glucose Tolerance: An Even Keel

Exercise after having your baby can help you improve your blood chemistry by improving your response to insulin and your glucose tolerance.[34,39] Insulin is a hormone your body secretes to transport energy from something you ate to where it needs to go in your body (the main destinations are muscles, fat, or your liver). Energy (food) comes in three forms: fat, carbohydrate (the simplest form is sugar, or glucose), and protein. Although insulin transports all three of these forms of energy, it is most sensitive to sugar (glucose). You can think of insulin as a shuttle that moves the energy where it needs to go. About 8–10 minutes after you eat a meal, you'll start to have the insulin shuttles arriving in your blood, ready to transport the energy. Their activity peaks after about 30–45 minutes.[42] After the insulin has transported all of the energy, you'll have a period of time when you have some insulin just loitering around in your blood. The more sugary your meal, the more insulin you'll have loitering around after the energy has been transported. During those periods of time you may feel tired or like you need a pick-me-up in the form of a sugary snack, which can begin a vicious cycle. You probably already know about this phenomenon—it's better known as a sugar rush followed by a crash. Keeping your insulin level on an even keel (without a spike in sugar or insulin) will help you to feel better throughout the day and reduce the urge to eat sugary snacks. That can be particularly helpful for women who experienced gestational diabetes mellitus (GDM). Women who experience GDM are at higher risk for developing type II diabetes, and exercise can be an important part of a prevention program. Exercise will help to smooth out the insulin/glucose ups and downs by improving the responsiveness of insulin to glucose and helping your body's response to the insulin. This will make you feel better throughout the day, and it will help to prevent diabetes in the future.

Bone Health

Breastfeeding is one of the best things that you can do for yourself and for your baby (you will read more details about how exercise affects breastfeeding in chapter 6), but it will result in a temporary decrease in your bone mineral density. Your bones will return to their baseline density after you finish breastfeeding and your period resumes,[39] but the temporary change in bone density requires careful progression with impact exercises (such as running). This program includes a detailed, gradual run progression and a jogging stroller run progression.

While some degree of caution while beginning impact exercises is necessary when you are breastfeeding, exercising will actually help to slow the bone density loss you will experience. Except for the time that you are pregnant and breastfeeding, up until you're about 30 years old, your bone mineral density will generally be increasing or staying about the same. Post-menopausal women lose 1–2 percent bone mineral density per year, and the breastfeeding mom will lose 3–9 percent of bone mineral density during two to six months (after stopping breastfeeding, bone density will return to your baseline values).[37] That's 1.5–9 times the amount of bone mineral density loss in one-sixth to one-half the time. The decrease in bone density occurs at the fastest rate during the first five months of breastfeeding. While the bone density loss associated with breastfeeding means that we need to be careful when progressing impact exercises, exercise will actually help us to maintain a higher bone density while breastfeeding compared to breastfeeding moms who don't exercise.

> **Slow the Bone Loss, Accelerate the Fat Loss**
> A recent 2009 study showed that new, exclusively breastfeeding moms who exercised six days per week (three days of core strengthening and weight bearing strength training plus three days of aerobic exercise) had significantly slower bone density loss five months after giving birth than those who did not exercise. As an added bonus, both groups lost weight (they were explicitly instructed *not* to go on weight-loss diets), but the group that exercised lost significantly more body fat, and the non-exercising group lost significantly more lean body mass.[37]

Fatigue and Postpartum Depression

During the first few months after giving birth, it's common to feel fatigued, both mentally and physically. Some mothers even experience postpartum depression. If you think that you may be experiencing postpartum depression (PPD), if you think you may harm yourself or your baby, or that you are unable to care for your baby, you need to seek professional help immediately. Call your doctor, visit your local emergency room, or visit www.postpartum.net for help. If you are feeling fatigued, let your doctor know so that he or she can make sure there isn't another underlying medical reason causing the fatigue.

Postpartum Depression

Exercise can help to prevent PPD, and it can be part of a program to help recover from PPD. Exercise should be only one part of your recovery program, and I want to stress that if you think you may be experiencing PPD, even to a small degree, you need to get help from your doctor. Mention to your doctor that you are considering an exercise program and have your doctor decide if, how, and when exercise should be a part of your recovery program.

Postpartum Depression Statistics

If you are experiencing symptoms of depression, you are not alone. Some studies show that 30 to 50 percent of women experience some feelings of depression during the first few months after giving birth.[43] During the second, third, and sixth months after giving birth, the numbers are the highest.[44] A 2007 study revealed that among American mothers, 11–15 percent experience mild depression, and 17–23 percent experience moderate to severe depression. Those in the lowest income bracket (< $25,000 per year) and younger moms (18–24 years old) have the highest rates of depression. Those who work full time are more likely to have mild depression but less likely to have moderate to severe symptoms.[43] Exercise can help with these symptoms by improving your general self-esteem and mood, decreasing your fatigue, and lowering your feelings of anxiety.[34]

In the general mom and non-mom population, exercise can reduce symptoms of anxiety and depression, and this effect is more potent among women compared to men. Rates of PPD are lower among moms who exercise compared to those who don't.[34] Recent research out of Australia has shown that exercising regularly on your own or even just attending a once weekly hour and a half exercise class has a good chance of helping your mood and decreasing your risk for PPD.[45] A little exercise can go a long way in helping your mood and risk for PPD. A study of moms in Japan showed that regular exercise helped to improve their energy level and self-esteem. They also saw themselves as significantly more physically capable than their non-exercising peers.[46] Exercise takes up such a small part of your day, but its effects are far reaching in every aspect of your life.

Fatigue

Anywhere from 44 to 95 percent of moms experience postpartum fatigue, or a feeling of being physically or mentally tired during the first year after having their baby.[47] If you have already had your baby, this probably does not surprise you. Actually, what surprises me is that there are 5 to 56 percent of moms reporting that they are not fatigued. They are either liars or harboring some secret I would like to get my hands on. At 12 months postpartum, 67 percent of women report severe fatigue.[48] If you are feeling drained, you're in good company, but unfortunately those feelings of fatigue may last until your baby's first birthday and beyond. Feeling fatigued is not fun, and even worse, fatigue can contribute to postpartum depression, and it can negatively affect your relationship with your baby even if you're not experiencing depression.[48] Fortunately, exercise can help with fatigue as well.

There is a difference between feeling fatigued and feeling sleepy. If you just feel like you don't have the get-up-and-go that you normally do, or if you feel like you're just not able to concentrate as well no matter how much sleep you get, that's fatigue. You can certainly be both sleepy and fatigued, but when you know you've gotten enough sleep and you're simply feeling physically or mentally sluggish, that's more likely fatigue. If you know you're not getting the amount of sleep you need, you're likely feeling sleepy. Those are just a few examples—only you will know the difference between fatigue and sleepy for your body, and you or your doctor need to make that call. When you are truly feeling sleepy (perhaps after being up half the night), you need your rest. Sleep when your baby sleeps. Don't push through feeling sleepy—you need to be a mom to your baby more than you need to have perfect exercise attendance.

Fatigue can be mental or physical, and exercise can reduce both kinds of fatigue. Mental fatigue relates to difficulty concentrating or keeping focused on something. Physical fatigue has more to do with how much you feel like you can do and whether you feel like you're in good or bad physical condition. Although it might seem counterintuitive that exercise can make you feel less fatigued, more and more research is showing that exercise reduces both mental and physical fatigue in new moms throughout the world. Chances are if exercise is already a part of your life, you're familiar with this phenomenon. If you're feeling a little unfocused or sluggish, a brisk walk outside or a quick set of exercises can really give you the boost you need to get through your day. Now there's an emerging body of research that is verifying this effect for new mothers.

When you are simply feeling fatigued, just 60–120 minutes of exercise *per week* can significantly decrease your feelings of physical fatigue (get-up-and go) as well as mental fatigue (difficulty concentrating). This amount of exercise (about 10–15 minutes per day) will help to decrease feelings of mild to severe physical fatigue, and it will help to reduce feelings of mental fatigue as well (though it will have more of an effect on severe than mild mental fatigue).[48] A recent study in Taiwan showed that women who participated in just six to nine exercise sessions during the first three weeks after giving birth showed both decreased physical and mental fatigue.[47] Even just a short exercise session can help you to feel more energized and mentally refreshed for the rest of the day, so if you're feeling overwhelmed and fatigued, just commit to 15 or 20 minutes of exercise. You may even start to feel better and continue for a longer workout, and at the very least it will help you to feel more energized for the rest of your day.

Even if you've been committed to exercise your whole life, motherhood can add tremendous new challenges. You are on call 24 hours, 7 days a week. Time constraints, fatigue, and feeling guilty about doing something for yourself can all make it more difficult to get your workout in. Please remember that even a short workout can significantly benefit your mood and overall energy level, and that can have a fantastic effect on your ability to bond with your baby and your quality of life. If you are feeling fatigued or totally crunched for time, just make a short commitment. Don't even change into your exercise clothes—just get started with a few exercises and see where your workout goes. At the very least you'll be able to take a personal time-out and see mood and energy level benefits from a 15–20 minute mini-workout, and you might even be able to get your full workout done. Staying committed to exercise will help you to improve your functional abilities as a mom, improve your cardiovascular health and strength, and improve your blood chemistry and bone health. And don't feel guilty. Making an exercise program a regular part of your life now will give it staying power as a daily habit, which will benefit you and your family for decades to come by decreasing your risk for chronic disease, becoming overweight or obese, and lengthening your life expectancy. As you'll see in the next chapter, it will help your baby to develop the same types of habits with all of the same benefits for his or her life too. It's truly one of the best gifts you can give your baby.

CHAPTER 5
Benefits of Mom's Exercise for Baby

When my son was a newborn, I kept hearing that exercise was one of the best things I could do for my baby. I liked hearing that because it made me feel good about taking some time each day to do something for myself. I could do something for myself, but I would also be helping my baby. What could be better? Yet I had this nagging question as I exercised while my baby napped: Is it really helping him if I'm out here doing exercises in the living room while he's sleeping?

Our generation is facing a health crisis because of the soaring rates of overweight and obesity. Our children are facing the same crisis, but it's more sinister for them because they're kids—they're babies who don't know that too much TV could be bad for them, whether broccoli or chocolate cake is a better food choice (heck, they don't even know what a food choice is), or the first thing about the importance of exercise. If they become overweight or obese at a young age, they will have a monstrous uphill battle ahead of them, and remember—they're only little. It starts with us to help them slay this nasty dragon and truly to save their lives.

Because of the chronic diseases associated with overweight and obesity such as type II diabetes, cardiovascular disease, and certain types of cancer, overweight and obesity are overtaking smoking as the number one killer in America.[49] Not only is the overweight and obesity crisis a killer, but it can negatively impact their day to day lives by increasing their risk for developing bone and joint problems, sleep apnea, and emotional or psychological problems associated with stigmatization.[50] The current generation of children may not live longer than their parents, and it's because of the overweight and obesity crisis.

We can help them to fight this problem by teaching them about good nutrition from an early age (including starting with breast milk) and by instilling in them an active lifestyle from the very beginning. Our focus in this book is the physical activity part of the equation. To instill an active lifestyle, there are three steps we can take. First, get yourself in shape and keep it up. Second, be active with your child. Third, be present (not just in the physical sense, but really *be* there) for their physical or athletic endeavors.

Step 1: Get Yourself in Shape and Keep it up

Getting yourself in shape and keeping it up is important for your baby's future for three main reasons. First, your body composition and activity levels are predictors of your baby's future risk for becoming overweight or obese. In fact, during the first three years of his or her life, *your* BMI is more predictive of your baby's future body composition than his or her own BMI. Here are some numbers: a one to two year old with at least one obese parent has almost three times the likelihood of being obese as an adult compared to a one to two year old without either parent obese.[51,52] In children under three years old, the key predictor for the child's risk for becoming obese is the *parents'* BMI. Between the ages of three and nine, both the parents' BMI and the child's BMI are predictors of future obesity, and after the age of nine the child's BMI becomes the most predictive factor of adult obesity. Overall, a child under the age of ten has more than double the risk of becoming obese if he has just one obese parent compared to a child without an obese parent.[51]

Second, your activity level sets an example that your little one is likely to mirror. If you're active, your little one is likely to become active. If you are pretty sedentary, your little one will be too. If you watch a lot of TV, guess what? So will your little one. This parental mirroring has been studied in great detail recently, using questionnaires, pedometers (step counters), and accelerometers that can measure how fast you're moving whether you're walking or standing in one place loading groceries into the car.

It turns out that 73 percent of the time, children's physical activity level mirrors that of their mom, and 67 percent of the time it mirrors their dad's level of activity.[53] The more steps you take during the day, the more steps your children will take during the day. This is true for dads too, just to a lesser degree.[53] Some research shows a stronger relationship between the mom and son's number of steps,[53] and some research shows a stronger relationship between the mom and daughter's number of steps,[54] but there is a consistent strong relationship between the number of steps a parent takes each day and the number of steps the children take per day. That relationship is consistently strongest between the mom and her children, regardless of the child's gender, and tends to grow stronger as the children age.[54]

Your Activity Level Matters

A study in New Zealand used accelerometers to measure activity levels in children, then tried to match that data with lots of other factors, including the child's age, gender, BMI, and waist circumference as well as the parents' BMI, waist circumference, and physical activity level. The researcher also looked into TV watching restrictions, parental encouragement of physical activity, amount of time parents spent being active with their children, and number of times per week the children went to a park, playground, or beach with their parents. The only two factors that affected the children's moderate to vigorous physical activity levels enough to reach statistical significance were the parents' activity level and the age of the child (older children were more active, but that could be because of the accelerometer's ability to pick up more movement with the older kids' more advanced motor skills).[55]

Third, your exercise habits establish a family culture of exercise that has a good chance of becoming internalized by your baby and lasting a lifetime.[56] Overall, between zero and five years old[56] are the most important years for instilling a culture of exercise, and the effects will begin to show at about three or four years old.[34] Children aged four to seven with active moms are twice as likely to be physically active as four to seven year olds without active moms.[54] Healthy exercise and activity habits that begin during childhood tend to last into adulthood. Children who come from sedentary families are more likely to be sedentary as adults. Children who have good overall strength, flexibility, and fitness are likely to keep those attributes in adolescence and into adulthood. Kids who participate in sports are more likely to participate in sports as adults, and research shows that it is especially important to reinforce an active way of life during transitional periods such as transitioning from elementary to middle school and during puberty.[57] During times of change, it's important to keep healthy and stress-relieving habits such as movement and activity a part of their daily routines.

In the first years of your baby's life, you have a golden opportunity to make activity and movement a core aspect of daily life from the very start. Making your own exercise a priority during the first years of your baby's life gives you the ability and energy to incorporate movement and activity into the fabric of your baby's daily life, and that will stick with them as they grow up. The example you set by just being physically fit and prioritizing exercise teaches them that it's important to be active. The environment that you create by making exercise a part of your family's daily routine makes it easy and natural for them to become athletes too.

Step 2: Be Active with Your Child

What does it mean to be active with your child? To your little one, exercising with them means moving with them in the way they like to move. When your baby is a newborn, being active together means doing tummy time together and playing together in the baby floor gym. When your baby is crawling, being active together means getting down on the ground with them and exploring the house together. Toddlers want to jump and dance and run. Being active together with a toddler means getting silly together, dancing, jumping, and exploring to your hearts' content.

Getting your workout done in order to be a good role model and being active with your baby don't necessarily happen at the same time. It can be challenging to get your own workout done in a way that allows you to take a mental break, get a tough workout done, and at the same time make it a fun experience for your baby. Usually that means that your exercise time happens while your baby sleeps or is spending quality time with dad or another care provider. You can use your workout time to take a mental timeout, refresh your body, energize your spirit, and get ready for an action-packed day with your little one.

If you have a baby that loves stroller rides, great weather for being outdoors, and a selection of stroller-ready workouts, you can take your baby along for some fresh air and scenery while you exercise. (A stroller run progression is in Appendix C.) If you have a stroller group class that meets near your home, it's certainly worth a try. These groups can provide challenging workouts as well as support networks for new moms. Many of these groups meet at a local park so the little ones can play after class, which is a wonderful way to get some outdoor time for both of you. You are setting a positive example by incorporating exercise into your day, and more importantly, by playing together at the park afterwards you're being active with your child. If you don't have a stroller group class within a reasonable distance from your home, you can do a stroller workout from home. You don't have to be restricted to cardio workouts with your stroller, either. You can always bring a set of light dumbbells along and stop every half-mile to do two to three exercises (exercises like squats, lunges, and bent-over rows are great examples) if you need to incorporate some resistance training. When you get home, follow your workout up with a movement-centered indoor activity for your child or backyard play. If you fit exercise into your schedule when your baby is young and time is scarce, it will have staying power as your schedule and family grow and become more complex.

We can learn a lot about how important it is to be active with your child through studies that examine how strongly babies, toddlers, and preschool children mirror our activity levels depending on the time of day or day of the week. Research out of the UK has shown that preschoolers most strongly mirror their mom's activity levels during the weekdays, especially among children who were at home for more of the time (not in school or day care). While working moms tended to be more sedentary (since they often had desk jobs), the relationship between their activity level and their child's activity level was not as strong, since their child was at school or day care while they were working.[58] So the more the mom and preschool-aged child were together during the weekdays, the more closely their weekday physical activity levels correlated.

Overall, the more time you spend with your child, the more his or her activity level will mirror yours, and your child's activity level will most closely mirror your activity level during the time that you spend together.

Active Together Time
Studies on older kids have shown similar results. A recent study conducted in the US of 9 and 10 year olds showed that children whose parents were more active tended to be more active and those with less active parents tended to be less active. The relationships were strongest during the times of day that parents are typically with children of that age, such as after school and during the weekends, and the strongest relationships were mother-daughter and father-son. The child's physical activity level mirrored both mom and dad's activity level, and when both parents were more physically active, that had an even stronger effect on the child's physical activity level than just one active parent.[59]

Step 3: Facilitate and encourage your child's interests in movement and sports

If you are determined to create an environment rich with activity and movement that encourages an active lifestyle for your child, adding lots of TV to the mix can be destructive. Information is widely publicized and available to show the counterproductive effects TV has on infants' brain development. It's also counterproductive for their long-term physical health too. Believe it or not, 17 percent of children 0–11 months old watch more than *2 hours* of TV per day. Between the ages of 12–23 months, that number more than doubles and 48 percent of children watch more than 2 hours of TV per day.[56] The American Academy of Pediatrics recommends that for children under the age of two, screen time should be altogether discouraged, and for children older than two, entertainment screen time should be kept to less than one to two hours per day.

Inactive Together Time

Just as active time correlates between parents and children, so does inactive time. Your children will mirror the amount of time you spend watching TV. Research in the UK of 10–11 year olds showed that the relationship between parent TV-watching time and child TV-watching time is strong for both girls and boys. In that study, girls were 4 times as likely to watch over 4 hours of TV per day if their parents watched between 2 and 4 hours of TV. Boys were 10 times as likely to watch over 4 hours of TV per day if their parents watched over 4 hours of TV per day.[60]

How does TV watching make it harder for children to be active? Most obvious, while they're watching TV, they're not doing anything active. Second, they're more sleep deprived, and third they're eating more. Not only are they mindlessly munching in front of the TV, but they're exposed to advertisements for fast food and junk food.[61] A worldwide study using surveys of over 77,000 children (ages 5–8) in 18 countries and over 200,000 adolescents (ages 12–15) in 37 countries confirmed the suspicion that watching more TV directly correlates with a higher BMI. For every category, boys and girls, children and adolescents, throughout the world, more TV meant higher BMI. The TV watching was broken into categories by time (1–3 hours, 3–5 hours, or more than 5 hours per day), and at every increasing time increment, BMI increased, and that was true for boys and girls, children and adolescents. Even in the lowest TV-watching category (1–3 hours per day) risk for overweight and obesity increased by 10–27 percent for all of the children and adolescents.[61] Sometimes it is tempting to have the TV on to distract your little one while you get things done (including a workout) or to just have some background noise, but this can be very counterproductive for your child. In creating your healthy active family environment, it is a good idea to minimize screen time, even tiny screens on smart phones or tablets.

When your little one is a baby, you can support his or her involvement in physical activity by being present—getting down for tummy time to be physically present and putting away distractions like your smart phone and turning off the TV to be mentally present. As your baby turns into a child and then a teenager, supporting physical activity will look more like setting TV restrictions, being active with them, and providing logistical support for their activities (such as driving them to practice).[62,63] A recent study of 193 children in the Midwest showed a direct correlation between the moms' encouragement of physical activity and the child's actual physical activity (average age was nine and a half), and the more the mom encouraged physical activity, the lower the child's BMI.[64] More and more research is emerging to support what is already intuitive—if we encourage and support our children's physical activity, they will have healthier bodies and more active lifestyles.[65] [62–64]

The role you play in ensuring an active lifestyle for your baby will change as the years go by. You'll do hurried workouts during naptime, get down on your belly for tummy time together, dance and run together, set limits for the TV, be the biggest fan at little league games, and drive them to practices and events all over the county—maybe even the country. As your role changes over the years, three things should remain: you remain consistent with your own exercise commitment, you participate in activities with them (whether it's tummy time or playing catch or simply going on walks together), and you support them by being present, minimizing counterproductive influences (like TV), and encouraging them every step of the way.

CHAPTER 6
Breastfeeding and Exercise

As a physical therapist, I have found myself time and again in complete awe of the capabilities of the human body. Breastfeeding knocks my socks off. Through breastfeeding, we have the ability to provide our babies with a perfect source of nutrition that is balanced with exquisite precision and based upon their individual and ever-changing needs. If you are breastfeeding your baby and you are worried about the effects of exercise on the quantity or quality of your milk, or if you are worried about how breastfeeding will affect your weight loss, let me give you an update of what the latest research has found on this topic. I want you to know the basics about how your body prioritizes your energy balance during breastfeeding and what that means for your baby and you. You will find that exercise and breastfeeding are actually quite complementary, and they are some of the very best things you can do for your baby and for yourself.

Concern that exercise will deplete milk supply is so common that it has been the target of repeated research studies in the past several decades. Consistently, research studies show that regular exercise does not deplete the volume of milk you produce, nor does it have a negative effect on the nutrient composition of your milk.[39,41,66,67] In fact, some studies even found that exercising women produced slightly *more* milk (not statistically significantly more, but slightly more) than non-exercising women.[67] How is that possible? If you have a lower amount of body fat, your milk will be lower in fat.[68] Since it's lower in fat, it has fewer calories per fluid ounce, and your body makes more in order to supply your baby with enough calories. Therefore, if you have lower fat content in your milk, you may make slightly more.

Ask your doctor for individual guidance if any of the following are true for you. Your doctor knows your individual history and situation, and she can provide you with the help that you need, including, if needed, an appointment with a lactation consultant or dietician.
  ➤ Your baby has any kind of special needs
  ➤ You think that you may need to go on a special diet to help you lose your pregnancy weight for health reasons
  ➤ You have a low BMI of less than 18.5
  ➤ You have struggled with nutrition and weight loss or gain in the past
  ➤ Your baby is not gaining weight as he or she should
  ➤ You are planning to train for any form of athletic competition during breastfeeding
  ➤ You have questions about how your diet and exercise plan could affect your baby's growth and development

Overall, research shows that regular exercise and a good diet will not negatively affect your breast milk, but we need to establish some boundaries here. If you have a BMI under 18.5, you are at risk for a decrease in milk supply if you are not careful to balance your input (amount of food you eat) with your output (daily activities + exercise). If you fall into that category, you need to see your physician, a lactation consultant, or a dietician to help carefully manage your input.[67] If you add calorie restriction to your post-pregnancy plan, please do so under the care of a physician, lactation consultant, or dietician. Your body's first priority is to keep your baby thriving, and if you severely restrict your diet to fewer than 1500–1800 kcal per day, there's some research that indicates you'll start to have hormonal shifts that will initially produce an increase in milk to protect your baby from perceived impending starvation followed by a decrease in supply.[66] For most women, however, a reasonable diet (certainly more than 1800 kcal per day) and exercise program will not result in a change in breast milk supply or nutrient composition.

For many breastfeeding women, it's not necessary to restrict calories in order to lose weight after giving birth. Breastfeeding requires an additional 500–650 kcal per day,[40,67] which is an even higher demand than pregnancy.[68] You may feel very hungry when you're breastfeeding, and you might even find that you're eating larger portions and adding snacks, especially in the beginning. If you're really in tune with your appetite, you'll notice surges in your hunger as your baby reaches new milestones, like when your baby starts to crawl.

There are basically two ways to meet the added energy demand of breastfeeding. You can eat more, or you can do less. Both of these methods will come naturally, without you even having to think about it—you just have to listen to your body. As a whole, women generally do some of both: 56 percent of the added calories come from eating more and 44 percent are conserved by doing less, and most often there is a net burn of body mass. In the second month after giving birth, exclusively breastfeeding women average a loss of 15.7 grams of fat per day.[68] For most women who aren't consciously dieting, that translates to an average of 0.44 to 1.77 pounds of weight loss per month during the first 6 months (that's after the initial rapid weight loss in the first few days and weeks after giving birth) and about 0.22 to 0.44 pounds per month in the second 6 months.[68]

Diet, Exercise, and Milk Supply

A study published in the prominent *New England Journal of Medicine* in 2000 followed overweight breastfeeding moms from week 4–14 after giving birth. Half exercised for 45 minutes 4 times per week and dieted (under strict guidance and still consuming more than 1800 kcal per day), and the other half did neither. At the end of 10 weeks, there was no difference in the babies' weight gain or length growth between the two groups. The moms were different, though, with the diet and exercise moms losing an average of 10.5 pounds and the do-neither moms losing an average of 1.7 pounds.[66] This study, published in 2000, was great news—it is possible for overweight moms to lose weight in a healthy way (through prescribed diet and exercise) while breastfeeding without negatively affecting milk supply.

Every woman is different when it comes to losing her pregnancy weight after giving birth, but research has shed some light on some generalities. Exclusively breastfeeding for the first six months is actually the best way to continue to lose weight after having a baby. Research studies about breastfeeding generally divide moms into three categories: exclusive breastfeeders, breast and bottle combination feeders, and formula feeders. In the first three months after giving birth, formula feeding moms lose the most weight, followed by exclusively breastfeeding moms, and last the combination-feeding moms. In the first three months, if you are exclusively breastfeeding, your body will preserve your fat stores as a way to provide extra insurance for the baby—if something should happen to your food supply, you will be able to "burn the furniture" to continue to provide milk for your baby. After those first three months, exclusive breastfeeders start to lose more weight than both of the other groups of moms.[41,68] At six months, when solids are typically introduced, exclusive breastfeeders will have lost the most weight, followed by combination feeders, and lastly the formula-only feeders will have lost the least amount of weight (3–6 pounds less than the exclusively breastfeeding moms and 1.85 pounds less than the combination feeding moms).[40,68]

Moms who are breastfeeding lose weight at an even faster rate during months 9–12 of breastfeeding—there's a hormonal shift at that point when your baby becomes more mobile and needs more calories, and that allows you to really tap into your fat reserves to feed your baby. These trends continue in the long-term; by one year, moms who are still breastfeeding are more likely to have returned to their pre-pregnancy weight, and formula feeding moms tend to stay at about 4 percent above their pre-pregnancy weight by their baby's second birthday.[68]

During the first few months of breastfeeding, exercise isn't likely to cause you to lose any more weight than you would lose if you weren't exercising. Your body's main priority is to feed your baby, so if you're exercising, you'll either be hungrier and eat more or reduce your activities throughout the rest of the day (even subconsciously) in order to protect your milk supply. A 1994 study illustrated this beautifully by researching breastfeeding moms of newborns for 10 weeks and assigning half of them to an exercise program. When the only difference between breastfeeding moms was the addition of exercise without any advice about diet, the exercising moms didn't lose more weight than the non-exercising moms. The exercising moms naturally ate more, and in the second five weeks of the study, they started to decrease their daily around-the-house activities on their own. The differences between the groups were an increase in their maximal oxygen uptake and a higher protein content in the milk of the exercising moms.[69]

Some women need more than just exercise and breastfeeding to lose their pregnancy weight (some women even gain weight while breastfeeding), and for those women the best strategy to lose weight is a combination of a restrictive diet (again, discuss with your doctor first), regular exercise, and exclusive breastfeeding for the first 6 months.[40] If exclusive breastfeeding for the first 6 months isn't an option, exclusive breastfeeding for even just the first 12 weeks can result in long-term benefits for you by preventing excess weight gain in the future.[40] Dieting alone can help you to lose weight, but the results tend to be a loss of lean mass instead of fatty mass. You're interested in losing the fatty mass, not the lean mass. If you add exercise to diet while you're breastfeeding, your body will burn your fat as a buffer to protect the breast milk supply.[69]

When you're breastfeeding, your body's mission isn't your weight loss—it's your baby's nutrition, and to sustain your milk supply, your body operates in a precise, priority-driven way. Here's a run-down of your body's priorities. First, feed the baby by having mom eat more. If that's not possible, option two is to use mom's fat stores. If fat stores are low, option three is to decrease mom's energy expenditure with all other activities. If that's already in place and still more energy is required to feed the baby, your body will improve your energy efficiency for all tasks. If you're out of options, the last resort will be a decrease in milk supply.[68] The best way to showcase this priority-driven ability to maintain milk supply is to examine the lives of women who can't go to Trader Joe's for more food or put their feet up to relax during their baby's nap time. Typically, if we are breastfeeding and on a diet, we'll naturally do less throughout the day. If we're breastfeeding and exercising, we'll naturally eat more. But what about women who don't have those options? Research from Gambia to Nepal to the Phillipines has shown that breastfeeding mothers have an amazing ability to maintain milk supply even in the face of subsistence farming, where there is no wiggle room for eating more or doing less.

Breastfeeding Around The World

Studies in Gambia and the Northwest Amazon of subsistence farming communities (where everybody has to work in order to have enough for everybody to eat, and nothing is left over to sell) showed that women who were breastfeeding took on less taxing jobs in order to maintain their energy balance.[68] Women in rural parts of the Philippines typically don't see significant post-pregnancy weight loss (beyond the initial sharp drop in weight) until after 10–14 months of breastfeeding. They are undernourished as a group, so they don't have the option of increasing intake or using mom's fat stores—their only options are to decrease activity or increase efficiency with their activities in order to preserve milk volume, and during the first 10–14 months, that means staying at a fairly stable weight.[70] For women in rural Nepal, the season determines a lot: physical activity, food intake, work output, and nutritional status. The Tamang are a people in the foothills of the Himalayas who live at an altitude of over 6,000 feet and have no electricity or medical facilities, and they have a full day of walking to get to a market or road. Recent studies of these women showed that they made small adjustments in their output by cutting back on outdoor work during the more work-intensive seasons. This resulted in about a 50 kJ/day difference for pregnant women and about a 1000 kJ/day difference for breastfeeding women during the work-intensive seasons.[71] With these studies, we can really see the body's ability to shift input and output (without any other variables like exercise or trips to the grocery store) in order to maintain the balance necessary for maintaining milk supply.

There are a few temporary changes in your breast milk that you should be aware of when you are planning your regular exercise program in conjunction with your feeding schedule. Some babies are sensitive to the change in taste of breast milk right after exercise, and others don't seem to mind at all. There is also a slight decrease in some antibodies during the first 10–30 minutes after exercise. Research of breast milk after exercise shows that there is an increase in lactic acid in the milk (anywhere from a 36 percent increase after submaximal exercise to a 650 percent increase after exercising to exhaustion) 10 minutes after exercise. That lactic acid can affect the taste of the milk, but the reviews from the babies in these studies are mixed. For some, it matters less how much lactic acid was in the milk and more whether they were fed with an eye dropper (ick! Whose idea was that?) versus a familiar bottle.[39] For others, breast milk was less palatable in the first 10–30 minutes after exercise.[69]

Though babies wouldn't taste it, the increase in lactic acid can also *temporarily* cause a decrease in immunoglobulin A concentration (an important antibody for protecting your baby from infection) in the first 10–30 minutes following exercise.[41] Only your baby can be the judge of the taste of your milk, and you'll have to weigh all of these factors when determining the best time for a planned feeding after you exercise (that is, if your baby lets you make the choice).

Overall, your body has an amazing ability to balance intake and output in order to provide milk for your baby. Many women worry that exercise will cause their milk supply to decrease, but your body has several natural mechanisms to keep your milk supply up so long as you keep breastfeeding. If you are combination feeding, your body may not be as in tune with demand changes from your baby, and a consultation with a lactation consultant may be helpful. If weight loss is a priority for you for health reasons, and the average one-half to two pounds of weight loss per month after the initial rapid decrease in weight in the first few days and weeks after giving birth won't get you to reach your weight loss goal by the one-year mark, you may need to combine diet and exercise with breastfeeding, and that is done best under the guidance of your doctor, lactation consultant, and/or dietician.

CHAPTER 7
Common Postpartum Injuries

As a mom, you don't get sick days. You can't be sidelined by an injury. Each level of this program has built-in, research-backed exercises that are integral to preventing the most common mom injuries as well as recovering from the injuries that can carry over from pregnancy into the postpartum period. If you find yourself with posterior pelvic pain, low back pain, a separation in your abdominal muscles (diastasis recti), carpal tunnel, or foot pain that just hasn't gone away after you've had the baby, or if you develop "baby wrist" or upper back, shoulder, or neck pain in caring for your newborn, I'll show you a few tweaks for your program and self-treatment tips that can really help. I'll also give you some guidance on seeking help from a medical professional—who specializes in what and how to find them.

Back Pain

What is it?
Back pain can be general or pinpoint, it can be in the mid back, the low back, or the pelvis, and it can stay in the back or radiate to the buttocks or even down the leg to the foot. Overall, back pain is the most common musculoskeletal pain afflicting moms and those who care for babies and children under the age of four.[72] It is not uncommon for back pain to start during pregnancy, and when it does, it usually starts in the fifth or sixth month of pregnancy.[23] About half of pregnant women with back pain have pain in more than one spot, such as in the mid back, the low back, or in the pelvis, so the term "back pain" is a term for pain in a broad region of your body.[73] The most common location for back pain, including for pregnant women, is the low back, so low back pain will be our focus in this section.

How common is it?
If you experience low back pain while you are pregnant or caring for a little one, you are certainly not alone. It affects about half of all parents with children under the age of four.[72] Anywhere from 25 to 90 percent of pregnant women experience low back pain during pregnancy,[5,14,23,74] which is a huge range, but discrepancies aside, low back pain during pregnancy is common, and it can be severe and debilitating for some women. Of those with severe low back pain, 19 percent even decide not to have another baby because they are worried the pain could come back with another pregnancy.[23] Seven percent of pregnant women report their low back pain to be disabling during pregnancy.[75] The good news is that there are steps you can take to prevent and repair low back pain.

Can I reduce my risk of developing back pain?
There are a few ways to reduce your risk for developing back pain before becoming pregnant. If you are reading this section, it's likely that you already have back pain and you may have already had your baby, so knowing how to reduce your risk for developing back pain during pregnancy can be helpful for your next preg-

nancy, especially since a previous history of back pain is a risk factor for future back pain.[23] You have a lower risk for developing low back pain during pregnancy if you are more fit before getting pregnant, even if you only exercise 45 minutes per *week*, and you're also at lower risk if you remain active during your pregnancy.[5,23] Some factors that increase your risk for low back pain that aren't as easy for you to control are sleep problems and your work situation. If you aren't sleeping well or if you're working part time in a physically demanding job, you're at a higher risk for developing low back pain.[23,73] Consistent exercise, then, is one of the best things you can do to take control and help prevent back pain in a future pregnancy.

What's the natural course of low back pain?

Low back pain that starts during pregnancy often lingers for about 1–3 months after giving birth,[75] but in about 40 percent of women, the pain can last for 18 months,[73,75] and for about 10–20 percent of women, the pain can even last for 2–3 years or longer.[74] You can decrease your risk of lingering pain by returning to a healthy weight (though not necessarily your pre-pregnancy weight) by 6 months after giving birth and strengthening your core, including your pelvic floor muscles as well as your abdominal muscles.[75]

What causes low back pain?

For years and years medical care providers sought to identify the anatomical structure responsible for a person's low back pain in order to guide their treatment plan—if you can find the culprit, you can fix the problem, right? It hasn't been quite so straightforward. We can truly and correctly identify a structure in the low back causing pain (such as a joint, a ligament, a particular muscle, or a disc) less than 10 percent of the time.[76] There are lots of different structures in the low back, and they physically overlap and refer pain to a variety of intersecting locations, creating a very confusing environment. On top of that, there are so many structural layers overlapping one another that a particular structural problem might not be painful at all—the pain may come from another structure that appears fine on imaging studies. In that case, treating the "problematic" structure would have us missing the mark entirely. Well over half (62 percent) of people with no back pain at all, for example, will have MRI findings that show serious disc problems such as protrusions, extrusions, and herniations in their back.[77] Over time and by using research, we have learned to ask better questions, use imaging studies only when they are truly helpful (imaging studies that show a problem where there is no pain can actually be harmful), and classify patients according to how to help them get better rather than by what structure is causing the problem.

Determining the biomechanical cause of low back pain among pregnant women is likewise complicated and fairly inconclusive. In examining the cause of low back pain among pregnant women, there's a lot of speculation—it could be the rapid weight gain, the shift in the center of gravity coupled with the weakness of the abdominal muscles, the low back muscles that just can't keep up with the demand of carrying the new load without any help from the abs, the increased mobility of the hips and pelvis that create an unstable base for the spine, or the change in the arch of the low back. The cause could be hormonal or even vascular. The results of the research investigating these causes have been unable to find one silver bullet cause of back pain during pregnancy.

When there is a common problem such as low back pain and many possible causes, it's often because the cause is different for different groups of people—some pregnant women may have low back pain because of weight gain, some because of weakness, some because of increased mobility, and some because of an increased arch in their low back.[5,23,74] Nobody knows for sure what causes low back pain during pregnancy, but researchers have begun to look for patterns to help get a better picture of what might help pregnant patients feel better. Recently researchers discovered that your ability to use your abdominal muscles to perform a sit-up while pregnant has little to do with your likelihood to have back pain, but pregnant women who have weakness in the outside of their hip (in the gluteus medius muscle) are six to eight times as likely to have low back pain as those who have strong outer hip muscles.[14] These clues can help redirect our efforts away from strengthening outer abdominal muscles and towards stabilizing the pelvis, including by strengthening your hip muscles.

How is it treated?

Frustrating as it is to find a cause for low back pain, medical care providers have begun to look at low back pain from a new perspective so that we can help people get better, since that's the goal, after all. We have found some answers by looking at common characteristics among people who get better and then classifying them according to the treatments that worked for them. For example, some people get better with hands on treatment, and others get better with core strengthening exercises. People within each group share some similarities with each other. Knowing the characteristics that are similar within the groups, we can classify patients according to these characteristics. Once we sort them into the treatment category that's most likely to be successful for them, we drastically increase their chances of getting better.[76,78-80]

Among the general population, we can generally classify people with low back pain into three treatment categories.[79] Some people need to be stabilized with core training, some people need to be mobilized with hands-on treatment and exercises specifically designed to improve their mobility, and some people need to do specific, directional movements for pain that is traveling into their buttocks or down their leg. At some point in their treatment program, those who need to be mobilized and those who need directional movements will need stabilization exercises too. New moms often fit into the stabilization category right from the start because of the increased flexibility and decreased core functioning during pregnancy and the postpartum period.[76]

The key to stabilizing your body with core training is learning to activate your core muscles in the right way, at the right time, and with the right amount of strength. Stabilization training is particularly effective if the diaphragm and pelvic floor exercises are integrated with the abdominal and back core training and the core training incorporates dynamic movements rather than simply static training.[19,75,81]

How this program can help:

Retraining and functionally stabilizing your hip muscles and your core team, including your pelvic floor, your deep abdominal muscles, your deep back muscles, and your diaphragm, are central to this exercise program. Fortunately for you if you have low back pain, this is precisely the technique that recent research has shown to be the most effective for getting rid of low back pain among new moms. The core drills at the beginning of each workout, the hip exercises, the planks, and the bird-dog series of exercises will be particularly helpful for you.

Tweaks and tips:

If you have back pain, focus a little extra on your core drill exercises at the beginning of each workout (see pages 71–74 for instructions), and add these to a few of your functional movements throughout the day. Do a core drill while you're standing before lifting the laundry basket or picking up your baby to retrain your body to fire your core the right way before functional movements (which a healthy back does without you having to think about it). Also, set aside 5–10 minutes each day, whether or not you're doing a workout that day, and do your core drill exercises without any interruptions so that you can really focus on getting the movement correct. Do the exercises slowly and precisely, stopping for breaks if you feel that you're just not getting the muscles to fire correctly.

What about a support binder or brace?

Many new moms looking for a solution to low back pain or just looking for a way to help reduce the size of their postpartum tummies turn to support binders and braces. Research shows that exercising your core muscles as a part of a physical therapy program is significantly more helpful at reducing low back pain than wearing a brace or binder. Wearing a brace or binder and doing physical therapy exercises to strengthen your core muscles is even more helpful at reducing the low back pain than doing either one alone,[19] with one problem. To refresh your memory, the pressure inside your abdomen is in constant flux when you're moving and functioning, and restoring a healthy core team involves using your diaphragm, your pelvic floor, and your abdominal muscles to keep everything in balance while you move. If you apply a brace or binder to your abdomen, that pressure has to go somewhere, just like if you're doing a bunch of static abdominal core contractions as your sole "core" training, and that "somewhere" is north towards your diaphragm and south towards your pelvic floor. That has the potential to put a lot of strain on your pelvic floor while it's trying to heal and may prevent your diaphragm-pelvic floor springboard from relearning how to operate correctly. So overall, while a binder or brace may help low back pain in the short term when it's combined with core training, it may cause a longer battle in the future for getting the whole core team to work together correctly again so that you can maximize function and performance and minimize your risk for further injury.

Seeking help from a physical therapist:

If your pain is just not getting better after a few weeks of strengthening your core and you would like to seek help from a medical professional, there are a few different kinds of physical therapists that can help you. In some states you may need a referral from your doctor to see a physical therapist, but in many states (and the list is growing) you can see a physical therapist without a referral—for your state rules check out http://www.apta.org/StateIssues/DirectAccess/. If your back pain is accompanied by pain that travels into your buttocks or down your leg, a physical therapist trained in the McKenzie Method may be particularly helpful to you. It often takes years to become McKenzie certified, but you can find a list of certified clinicians near you at http://www.mckenzieinstituteusa.org. If you can't find one near you, many therapists are in training to become certified, and a call to your nearest clinic can help track one down. If you need hands-on care or your movement feels restricted or stiff, a physical therapist skilled in manual therapy may be particularly helpful. The American Physical Therapy Association has a great "Find a PT" tool available on their website http://www.moveforwardpt.com/. Each therapist lists their focus areas, and you'll be able to find one that lists "manual therapy" if that's what you're looking for. Any physical therapist who specializes in orthopedics, manual therapy, sports physical therapy, or women's health will be able to help you with checking your core stability exercises and personalizing them for you and your situation, but if you have pelvic floor issues along with your back pain (which is common), you can use the same "Find a PT" tool to find a physical therapist who specializes in women's health.

When back pain needs immediate attention
You need to seek immediate medical attention from your physician if the onset your back pain is accompanied by:
- ➤ Sudden unexplained weight loss (> 25 pounds in 6 months, *and* more than could be explained by having your baby and the initial weight loss)
- ➤ A fever, chills, general feeling of illness that starts with the onset of your back pain or drenching sweating at night
- ➤ Loss of control of your bladder or bowel movements and/or have numbness in your upper inner thighs
- ➤ A personal history of cancer

Posterior Pelvic Pain

What is it?

Many people with posterior pelvic pain consider their pain to be low back pain, but it is actually a separate problem and treated somewhat differently. Posterior pelvic pain is pain at the back of your pelvis, and it's often worse with weight- or load-bearing positions, such as standing, sitting, walking, or stairs, regardless of the position of your back.[82] Posterior pelvic pain can best be distinguished from low back pain by its location (low back pain can travel into the pelvis, but posterior pelvic pain stays in the pelvis and does not travel up to the low back) and its presentation (a particular characteristic of posterior pelvic pain is its sensitivity to load bearing—being on your feet, walking, or even sitting down, while mechanical low back pain is more consistently associated with certain movements regardless of whether you're standing, sitting, or lying down). It is actually even tricky for clinicians to distinguish posterior pelvic pain from low back pain in the clinic during an exam, so if you have a particularly resilient case of pain in your lower back/pelvic region, it's best to have a professional take a look (more on that below).

How common is it?

About 16–50 percent of pregnant women develop posterior pelvic pain,[82,83] and for some women it can be disabling. Often, posterior pelvic pain is more incapacitating than low back pain.[23]

What are the risk factors for developing posterior pelvic pain?

Women who have had back or pelvic pain in the past or previous trauma to the pelvis are more likely to develop posterior pelvic pain during pregnancy. Researchers have looked into BMI, smoking, epidural anesthesia, maternal ethnicity, bone density, number of previous pregnancies, contraception use, time since last pregnancy, and fetal weight as possible risk factors, but none of these had anything to do with the risk of developing posterior pelvic pain.[83]

What's the natural course of posterior pelvic pain?

The good news about posterior pelvic pain is that it's likely to resolve on its own. Most of the time (one research report indicates 93 percent of the time)[83] it will resolve in the first three months after giving birth,[23,82] approximately 95 percent of women will get better by the six month mark, and approximately 98–99 percent of women will get better by the one year mark.[83]

What causes posterior pelvic pain?

We've yet to discover one specific cause of posterior pelvic pain in pregnant women. Some possible causes include poor control of the muscle firing sequence of pelvic muscles[6] or core team muscles,[82] altered joint mechanics at the pelvis, or increased or uneven side-to-side pelvic joint movement.[82] After an injury (such as low back pain or pelvic trauma, which are the two known risk factors for developing posterior pelvic pain during pregnancy), our bodies compensate for the injury by picking up substitution patterns. While you're injured, you avoid certain painful movements, but you still have to function, so you start substituting. When those substitution patterns continue, you start to develop things like the altered joint mechanics or changes to your muscle firing sequences or side-to-side asymmetries that we see among women with posterior pelvic pain. That's why it is so important after you've been injured or altered your mechanics to really retrain the muscles not only for strength but also for correct firing patterns—not only does that help you to get better but it also may decrease your risk for future injury.

How is it treated?

At first, the treatment goals for posterior pelvic pain are to decrease the pain so that you can get to work retraining your muscles. During a bout of posterior pelvic pain, your deep core muscles stop working like they should because of the pain, and with your deep core muscles not working like they should, you're unable to stabilize your pelvis, so the pain in your pelvis gets worse, and the cycle continues.[82] To help decrease the pain, you need to avoid things that would aggravate your pelvic joints, such as stairs if possible, standing on one leg, and any extreme movements of the pelvis or back[23]—such as a deep lunge stretch or standing with one leg on the ground and one knee in the car and twisting as you pull the infant seat out of the car. Instead, keep both feet in the same place if you can and work in small stages to get the infant seat out. Initially and simply, be kind to your pelvic joints and avoid positions that aggravate your pelvis. The next recommended step is to participate in individualized physical therapy program that targets proper pelvic, hip, and core muscle strengthening and activation patterns.[6,82,83]

How this program can help:

During this program, we'll start with basic core drill movements, activating your core muscles, including your pelvic floor in the correct order, before moving your arms and legs. As you improve, we'll incorporate more advanced limb movements to challenge your core, then add in multidirectional and multiplanar movements, eventually challenging your balance and rotation. All of these movements combined will progressively retrain your pelvic muscles and reteach the proper firing sequence so that it becomes second nature. We'll also work on your deep hip and pelvis muscles by first working on strengthening them in an isolated capacity, and then we'll incorporate dynamic and multiplanar movements to challenge them in more functional ways.

Tweaks and tips:

If any of the exercises reproduce your posterior pelvic pain, skip that exercise. If you are still experiencing posterior pelvic pain as this program progresses to lunges and exercises on one leg, skip the lunges and skip the single leg exercises. If your posterior pelvic pain is improving or it has resolved by the time you get to the lunges or exercises standing on one leg, proceed with caution for these exercises. Start with mini-lunges (only go down one quarter of the way, with a closer stance), and do the single leg standing exercises with no weights in your hands the first couple times you do the exercises, and then add weight very gradually only if it isn't painful. If you're seeing a physical therapist for your posterior pelvic pain, show him or her what you're doing in this program, and he or she can help you decide how to tweak your exercise program specifically for you as you heal.

Seeking help from a physical therapist:

If you're having posterior pelvic pain, you can get tailored exercises specifically for you and your pelvic mechanics from a physical therapist. You can use the American Physical Therapy Association website at http://www.apta.org/StateIssues/DirectAccess/ to find out if your state requires a physician referral to see a physical therapist. You can use the "Find a PT" tool on their Move Forward website at http://www.moveforwardpt.com/ to find a physical therapist to help you. Particularly helpful for posterior pelvic pain are orthopedic, sports, manual, and women's health physical therapists.

Incontinence

What is it?

Incontinence is the word we use to describe what's happening when you leak urine or have a fecal accident. Incontinence often has to do with a pelvic floor problem, especially after childbirth (the pelvic floor muscles are often either too weak, firing late or incorrectly, or overactive). Pelvic floor problems can show up in many ways, including as incontinence (probably the most obvious symptom to you), pelvic organ (uterine) prolapse, pain with sex, posterior pelvic pain, low back pain, and even more subtly as injuries in the arms or legs or even the jaw. That happens when the pelvic floor problem is disrupting the core firing pattern and setting off a chain of events that leads to poor body mechanics elsewhere.[84]

Incontinence is the most common and the most obvious of the pelvic floor dysfunctions. Urinary incontinence is more common than fecal incontinence, and there are many kinds of urinary incontinence, but the two most common types are stress urinary incontinence (SUI) and urge urinary incontinence.[12] Stress urinary incontinence happens when you have a sudden increase in your intra-abdominal pressure, such as when you sneeze, cough, or exercise, and your pelvic floor muscles just can't react in time or aren't strong enough, and urine leaks out.[85] Urge urinary incontinence happens when you have some kind of a trigger, such as running water or putting your key in the door, that makes you suddenly feel the urge to urinate.[86] Some continence problems are more subtle. You may have a problem with continence, for example, if you can't make it through the night without getting up to urinate or if you're urinating more than 7 times in a 24 hour period.[86]

How common is it?

About one quarter of all American women have some kind of pelvic floor dysfunction. Roughly 16 percent have stress urinary incontinence, 3 percent have pelvic organ prolapse, and 9 percent have fecal incontinence. Of women who had a vaginal delivery, 58% have some kind of pelvic floor disorder, as do 43 percent of those who had a C-section.[12] Among new moms as a whole, up to 34 percent have stress urinary incontinence.[85] Less than 1 percent of women who have never been pregnant have stress or urge incontinence.[87]

What are the risk factors for developing incontinence after giving birth?

The older you are when you have baby, the greater your risk for developing a pelvic floor disorder.[86,87] Likewise, the more babies you have, the higher your risk for having a pelvic floor disorder.[12] Your risk for developing incontinence after giving birth is higher following a vaginal birth than a C-section,[87] and if you have a long, active second stage of labor (the pushing stage) or if you deliver with the assistance of vacuum or forceps, your risk for developing incontinence (particularly urge incontinence following the use of vacuum or forceps) increases significantly.[12,87,88] Also, a previous vaginal delivery increases your risk for incontinence after future deliveries, even if you didn't have incontinence after the first delivery.[88] A third degree tear (a tear into the anus) and an episiotomy can increase your risk of developing incontinence, as can delivering a baby that weighs more than eight pounds.[86]

What's the natural course of incontinence?

Incontinence during pregnancy or early on in the postpartum period, even if it resolves on its own, can be a predictor for future pelvic floor problems if you don't take any action.[87] On the flip side, pelvic floor contractions, if done correctly, can be very helpful—73 percent of women treated with pelvic floor muscle exercises (supervised) have a complete resolution of incontinence, and 97 percent see improvement.[88] If you're having incontinence, or if you had incontinence when you were pregnant, you should consider seeing a women's health physical therapist (more on that below). Though temporary incontinence may be due to a transient, self resolving nerve injury from giving birth (this occurs in 38–42 percent of women during a vaginal delivery and may resolve within six months after giving birth),[12,87] seeing a women's health physical therapist can be enormously beneficial for helping to restore your pelvic floor and prevent future problems, from subtle pelvic floor problems to quality-of-life-altering, major problems.

What causes incontinence?

Giving birth is the most common cause of incontinence.[88] Your pelvic floor muscles don't just get stretched out and weakened during vaginal delivery, but during pregnancy as well, which is why even women who undergo C-sections are at risk for pelvic floor problems like incontinence.[88] The weight of the baby stretches the pelvic floor muscles and even changes some structural anatomy by changing the angle between the base of your bladder and your urethra, making the opening more of an oval than a circle. That creates a larger opening for your pelvic floor muscles to have to close to stop the flow of urine in their weakened state, making it doubly hard to maintain continence during and after pregnancy.[88] During some vaginal deliveries, the pelvic floor muscles are actually damaged and require sutures in the muscle to repair the tissue. This happens in third and fourth degree tears and with episiotomies. The new, remodeled, healed tissue is not as strong as the original tissue, and it can be challenging (though quite doable with work on your part) to get the muscles to fire like they should again. Damage to your pudendal nerve (the nerve that supplies the pelvic floor muscles) occurs 38–42 percent of the time, and as mentioned above, this usually self-resolves in the first six months after giving birth.[12] During the time that the nerve isn't working correctly, however, you can develop substitution patterns in your core that need to be addressed to help regain and maintain continence.

How is it treated?

Women's health physical therapists are physical therapists who focus on women's issues such as pelvic floor disorders and incontinence, and they are specially trained to evaluate and treat the pelvic floor. She will evaluate your pelvic floor muscle strength and function, then prescribe a treatment plan that may include muscle retraining (there are even pelvic floor weights you may be prescribed to train with), myofascial release, joint mobilization, biofeedback, and many other treatments depending upon your assessment.

As a general guideline, the National Institute of Health and Clinical Excellence recommends three months of pelvic floor strengthening exercises as the first line of treatment for stress urinary incontinence.[85,88] Those three months can be helpful only if you're doing the exercises correctly. Kegel exercises, first described by Arnold Kegel in 1948, are contractions of your pelvic floor muscles. If I were to verbally describe (or in this case, provide a written description) to you how to do a Kegel correctly and then send you on your way, you'd have a little lower than a 50/50 chance at getting that contraction correct. You would, in fact, have a 15 percent chance of doing the contraction in such a way that you'd be bearing down, which could cause further pelvic floor and incontinence issues for you,[86] so I'll describe the contraction for you, and then I'll tell you how to check it on your own.

To do a pelvic floor contraction, squeeze the muscles in your vaginal and anal area as if you're holding back gas without squeezing your buttocks together. You should feel tightening in area called your perineum between your vagina and anus. We'll cover two ways to check that contraction yourself: you can look with a mirror or you can feel for a contraction through thin clothing or underwear. Years ago, we used to consider it a good idea to check this contraction by trying to stop the flow of urine midstream. It turns out that not only can you stop the flow of urine by using a different set of muscles (substituting), thereby creating a false sense that you're getting the contraction right, but you can actually cause more problems for your urinary system and your pelvic floor muscles by practicing and checking this way.[86] You don't need to look or manually feel for a contraction every time you do your pelvic floor exercises, you just need to check when you're learning (or relearning) how to do the contraction correctly so that you know what right feels like before you proceed with the workout program. Even if you've done Kegels in the past, it's a good idea to look or manually feel for a contraction when you're relearning after giving birth.

It may be intimidating after giving birth to have a look at your nether-region, but if you are comfortable checking things out this way, lie on your back with a pillow under your hips and hold a mirror so that you can see the perineum (the area between your vagina and anus). When you do a pelvic floor contraction correctly, you should see your perineum or your anus pulling in towards your body.[86] If you see either of those two areas pushing out, you're bearing down.

To check the contraction through thin clothing or your underwear, lie on your side with a pillow between your knees (this is the easiest position for your pelvic floor to contract in). Feel for your perineum or anus, and when you do a contraction correctly, you should feel that area moving upward toward your head, or in other words, in toward your body.[86] If you aren't sure if you're getting this contraction correct, it's best to check the contraction with your OB or a women's health physical therapist before proceeding.

How this program can help:

During this program, you'll be doing pelvic floor contractions as a part of your core drill exercises at the beginning of each workout. You'll also be doing pure isolated Kegel exercises a few times a day. If you are able to get a correct pelvic floor muscle contraction by using one of the two methods listed above (look or feel), you'll be exercising in line with the recommended first step against incontinence: three months of pelvic floor retraining. If you are seeing a pelvic floor or women's health physical therapist, show her this program and double check with her to make sure each exercise you're doing compliments her program.

Tweaks and tips:

When you get started with each workout, spend a little extra time with your core drill exercises at the beginning of your workout. Make sure you get each contraction done well before moving on to the next one. Remember during your core drill exercises that your pelvic floor contraction should be at the end of your exhale, followed by your belly button pull, followed by relaxing both the pelvic floor and the abdomen to inhale. This is key. Lots of pelvic floor issues exist because of timing issues, and teaching your pelvic floor when to relax is a big part of retraining muscle sequence timing. If you're exercising with the video, just hit pause while you do your core drill exercises so that you're sure to take your time. When you get started doing your pure Kegel exercises throughout the day, do the exercises lying on your side or on your back so that your pelvic floor isn't fighting against gravity to contract. As you get better you can move into a sitting or standing position.

Seeking help from a physical therapist:

If you're experiencing incontinence that is affecting your quality of life or if you've tried to do the contraction on your own and you're either just not sure if you're getting it correct or if it doesn't seem to be helping, please seek out a women's health physical therapist. Don't ever feel embarrassed about an incontinence issue with your physical therapist. Many women's health physical therapists decided to specialize in women's health because of their own pelvic floor problems after giving birth, and they know the tremendous difference they can make in someone's quality of life by helping them recover from a pelvic floor dysfunction because at one point someone helped *them* to recover from a pelvic floor dysfunction. Some states require a consult from your physician to see a physical therapist, but many do not, and the number is growing. If you are incontinent, discuss the issue with your OB whether or not you plan to see a physical therapist. If your state allows for direct access to a physical therapist, you can make an appointment with or without a referral from your physician. You can check your state's direct access status at http://www.apta.org/StateIssues/DirectAccess/. To find a women's health physical therapist near you, you can use the "Find a PT" tool on the American Physical Therapy Association's Move Forward website at http://www.moveforwardpt.com/ to find a physical therapist to help you. You can look at each physical therapist's listed practice focus to find the words "women's health."

Diastasis Recti

What is it?

Your rectus abdominis, better known as your six-pack in your abdomen, has a fibrous cord running down the center (dividing the pack). When you're pregnant and your abdominal muscles stretch, your rectus abdominis separates at the center as this cord widens. That's totally normal, and separating at the center is part of how our body stretches to accommodate our growing baby. If that widening is more than 2.7 cm (about the width of two fingers) as measured at the level of the belly button, that's considered a problematic diastasis recti.[16] The recuts abdominis is an important member of your abdominal muscle team, and having diastasis recti problem can alter its functioning, putting you at risk for back pain and decreasing the stability of your pelvis and trunk.[16,89]

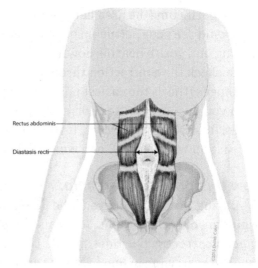

Figure 18. Diastasis recti

You can do a self check to see if you might have diastasis recti beginning three days after giving birth by lying on your back as if to do a crunch and placing three fingers in the center of your belly at the level of your belly button. Crunch up, just lifting your head off the ground until you *very first* feel the abdominal muscles move at the sides of your fingers. Stop there, and if you feel 2 or more fingers sink down into the space, that's a sign you may have diastasis recti.[89] Do the same check 4 cm above and 4 cm below your belly button. Keep checking, and you should feel that gap close up over the next eight weeks. If you suspect you may have diastasis recti problem as you near eight weeks, you'll have to get the actual diagnosis from a medical professional, but that test can give you a good clue about what may be happening.

How common is it?

During pregnancy, anywhere from 66 to 100 percent of women develop diastasis recti in the third trimester,[11,16] but the number decreases to just over 50 percent right after giving birth.[16]

What are the risk factors for developing diastasis recti?

The bigger your pregnant belly, the bigger chances developing diastasis recti—factors such as a larger baby or a large amount of amniotic fluid, carrying twins or more, or obesity all increase your risk for developing diastasis recti. Other factors related to your muscles themselves can increase the risk, such as weak abdominal muscles at the start of your pregnancy, overusing your abdominal muscles during the third trimester (doing lots of ab work while pregnant), intense pushing during childbirth, or pushing while holding your breath during childbirth.[89]

What's the natural course of diastasis recti?

If your diastasis recti is going to resolve on its own, that will usually happen in the first eight weeks after giving birth. After the first eight weeks, diastasis recti natural resolution hits a plateau.[16]

What causes diastasis recti?

At the same time your growing baby is stretching your abdominal muscles, your body is releasing hormones to loosen up your connective tissue.[16] That combination is often enough to separate the rectus abdominis muscle at the center.

How is it treated?

A 2014 systematic review, or a study of research studies, found very few high-quality studies investigating nonsurgical treatment options for diastasis recti. There are several authoritative tips available, but very few have actually been researched by comparing a group that participates in a program to a group that doesn't (the best version of this type of study is a randomized controlled trial). The research is particularly lacking in postpartum treatment of diastasis recti. To be clear, don't be discouraged. That doesn't mean that there isn't anything you can do, it just means very little has actually been studied.

The 2014 systematic review (study of research studies) of all studies about treatment of diastasis recti over the past 20 years found only one high-quality, randomized control trial conducted in 1999 in Brazil that showed significant reduction of diastasis recti.[90] The only problem with that study was that the exercises and treatment effects were conducted 6 and 18 hours post delivery, and that's it. Aside from that randomized controlled trial, the other studies were case studies—a description of what happened with one patient. Despite the lack of available research, we can look for some consistencies throughout the studies. The successful studies used a belly button pull contraction (see page 73) as a part of the routine to strengthen the transversus abdominis muscle, including the study of a woman who delivered her baby eight years earlier but still had a diastasis recti.[16] The transversus abdominis is key for reducing a diastasis recti because it is the deepest abdominal layer and functions like an internal corset. You can first strengthen the transversus abdominis muscle beneath it to help pull the rectus abdominis back together.

If you still have a diastasis recti of more than two centimeters eight weeks after giving birth, I recommend you see a physical therapist. A physical therapist will provide a hands-on evaluation and individualized treatment program. Since every woman's body is different and every diastasis recti will respond differently to abdominal muscle work, it's important to have a physical therapist guide you through an abdominal muscle re-training program.

How this program can help:

Learning how to retrain your core team, which includes your diaphragm, your pelvic floor, your transversus abdominis, and your deep back muscles, is central to this program. You'll start with the basic core drill contraction and gradually add more challenging and functional movements. This type of core work will help cinch that gap together, so that will be our focus.

Tweaks and tips:

Focus primarily on your transversus abdominis contraction (your belly button pull, on page 73). Avoid heavy use of the abdominal muscles during daily activities and avoid oblique crunches because of the risk of the oblique muscles pulling outward on the rectus abdominis muscle.[89] Also avoid exercises that are taxing for the rectus abdominis muscle, such as straight crunches, sit ups, or leg lowering exercises, unless you have received hands-on instruction from a physical therapist in a special way to do those exercises to help reduce the diastasis recti. In this program, skip the straight crunches, the oblique crunches (all varieties), the single and double leg lowering exercises, and all exercises performed in a plank-type position. You'll find modifications in the exercise charts for each level.

Seeking help from a physical therapist:

A physical therapist can provide you with evaluation and personalized treatment program for diastasis recti. You can use the American Physical Therapy Association website at http://www.apta.org/StateIssues /DirectAccess/ to find out if your state requires a physician referral to see a physical therapist (many states don't require a referral, and the number is growing). You can use the "Find a PT" tool on their Move Forward website at http://www.moveforwardpt.com/ to find a physical therapist to help you. Particularly helpful for diastasis recti are orthopedic, sports, manual, and women's health physical therapists.

Also be sure to check with your insurance company before your appointment. Even in states that allow for direct access to a physical therapist without a referral from a physician, some insurance providers require a physician's referral before they'll foot the bill.

Plantar Fasciitis

What is it?

Your plantar fascia is a long, thick, fibrous band along the bottom of your foot that goes from the front of your heel bone (calcaneus) all the way to the ball of your foot. It plays an important role in supporting your arch and making your foot dynamically rigid as you push off while walking or running. Runners, people who gain weight suddenly (such as pregnant women) or are obese, and people who spend a lot of time on their feet can irritate the plantar fascia right where the plantar fascia meets the calcaneus on the bottom of the foot.

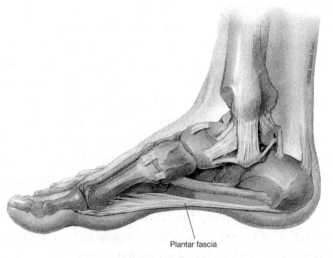

Plantar fascia

Figure 19. Plantar fascia

Irritation leads to pain and tiny microtears in the plantar fascia, which results in inflammation of the plantar fascia, AKA plantar fasciitis. Your body tries to repair these microtears by laying down clumps of collagen fibers over the microtears, usually at night.

Since nobody sleeps with their feet pulled back in a calf-stretch position, the attempted repair process happens with your plantar fascia on slack, or in a shortened position. When you step out of bed in the morning, your arch flattens, painfully disrupting all of the attempted healing that occurred through the night. For this reason, plantar fasciitis is most painful in the morning with the first few steps out of bed.

Typically the pain will improve with movement as the plantar fascia loosens up, but after a long day of pressure on an inflamed area and a fresh set of microtears, the pain will worsen again towards the end of the day. All of this tearing and attempted healing and re-tearing results in a vicious cycle.

How common is it?

About 10 percent of all adult Americans experience plantar fasciitis at some point in their lifetime.[91] There isn't any data available to show how common plantar fasciitis is among pregnant women and new moms, but theoretically it may affect new moms more than the general population because of the sudden weight gain and flattening of the foot during pregnancy[2], as well as the increased load postpartum as you carry your growing baby all day long.

What are the risk factors?

General risk factors for developing plantar fasciitis are sudden weight gain or obesity, high running mileage, decreased ankle flexibility, and prolonged standing throughout the day.[91,92]

What causes it?

There are two main factors at work in the development of plantar fasciitis. The first is the weight through your foot, and the second is the amount of time you spend putting weight through that arch, whether from walking, running, or standing. If the combination of your weight times the duration of standing, walking, or running is more than your plantar fascia can handle, you'll develop irritation where the plantar fascia meets the bone.

What's the natural course?

If left untreated, plantar fasciitis typically becomes chronic.

What's the non-operative treatment?

Treatment usually consists of three main options: stretch, support, or shoot (with a needle). The stretching consists of stretching your plantar fascia by crossing one ankle over your knee, then pulling your toes back to feel the stretch where you feel pain. You can add a little extra stretch to this by rubbing your thumb horizontally across your heel where you feel pain when you stretch. The other stretch is for your calf muscles—with your knee straight as well as with your knee slightly bent to get both major calf muscles. Supporting plantar fasciitis is achieved by using tape or orthotics (custom or off the shelf) to hold your arch in a supported position as it heals. Shooting can be in the form of injections or dry needling. Injections for plantar fasciitis include Botox to treat the muscles beneath the plantar fascia that may be problematic or corticosteroids to reduce the inflammation. Dry needling does not inject anything, but involves using a tiny acupuncture needle to release trigger points (knots) in your foot and lower leg muscles that can be causing or contributing to your pain. There are a few more treatments out there like breaking up the damaged tissue (if it has started to scar and calcify) with ultrasonic shock waves or spinning some of your blood down to mostly platelets, then reinjecting it into your foot to supercharge the healing process, but those are a little farther down the road if the other treatments aren't working.

How can this program help?

During this program, we'll be working on your deep foot and lower leg muscles that support your arch from Level 1 on. If those muscles are strong, they will take some of the onus off of the plantar fascia and help to provide it with some relief as it heals.

Tweaks and tips

Some immediate things you can do to treat your own plantar fasciitis are to stop walking in socks or barefoot at home, even (and especially) when you first step out of bed in the morning. You should even have arch support in the shower (arch-support flip flops work really well) or stand on the outside of your feet while showering. Supporting your arch will help maintain the healing process that goes on while you're resting. Wear arch-support shoes or slippers at home, and wear arch-support shoes throughout the rest of the day. If your shoes don't have arch support built in, you can buy a reasonable pair of arch-support insoles at a drugstore. You can also start the bottom of the foot stretching in the morning when you wake up and the calf stretching throughout the day.

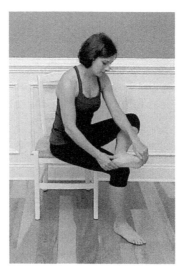

If you have a golf ball, stick it in the freezer or use a cold soda can to roll under your foot for some relief. You can also tape the plantar fascia on your own using a Cover-Roll Stretch Tape and Leukotape P (available at many online vendors such as Amazon and Drugstore.com).

My personal favorite treatment for my patients is to follow the instructions below for a custom, wear-anywhere plantar fascia support system. This taping technique was the technique used in a 2006 research study and it resulted in significant relief compared to stretching, placebo taping, or no treatment.[93] The tape usually works for about three days (though I've had patients keep it on for five days) before needing to reapply. You should feel relief as soon as you step down after putting the tape on—if it hurts worse, it's just not working. You can try reapplying the tape, but this isn't something that you should just keep pushing through to see results. You can wear the tape in the shower, and if you're wearing the tape, you can go barefoot because the tape is your arch support. Keep reapplying the tape until you feel better. This usually takes two to three weeks.

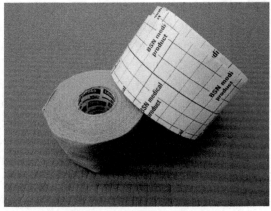

Leukotape and Cover-Roll Stretch Tape

Step 1: Cut four pieces of Cover-Roll Stretch Tape (white tape) and four pieces of Leukotape (brown tape). You can measure the pieces from the lower edge of your outer anklebone and below your heel to the lower edge of your inner anklebone. All eight pieces should be the same length.

White Tape First

Step 2: Place the first piece just below your outer anklebone around the back of your heel to just below your inner anklebone.

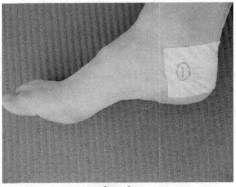

Step 2

Step 3: Place the second piece just below your outer anklebone and under your heel to just below your inner anklebone. The third and fourth pieces follow the same pattern, just farther down your foot, overlapping the piece before it by about half.

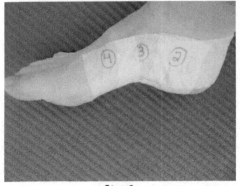

Step 3

56

Brown Tape Second

Step 4: Place the first piece just below your outer anklebone, then ***pull*** the tape as you bring it under your heel to attach just below your inner anklebone. Repeat for the next two pieces of brown tape, overlapping the piece before it by about half. Remember to ***pull*** with each piece.

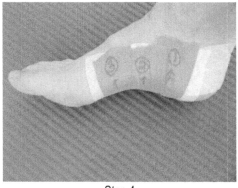
Step 4

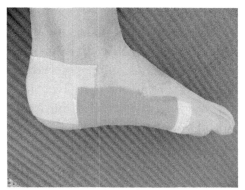
Step 4-2

Step 5: Place the final piece of brown tape just below your outer anklebone and pull it around the back of your heel to anchor it just below your inner anklebone.

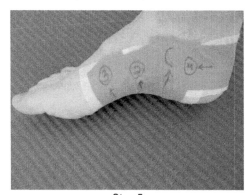
Step 5

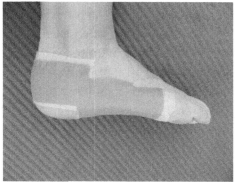
Step 5-2

Seeking help from a physical therapist:

A physical therapist can provide you with evaluation and personalized treatment program for plantar fasciitis. You can use the American Physical Therapy Association website at http://www.apta.org/StateIssues/DirectAccess/ to find out if your state requires a physician referral to see a physical therapist (many states don't require a referral, and the number is growing). You can use the "Find a PT" tool on their Move Forward website at http://www.moveforwardpt.com/ to find a physical therapist to help you. Particularly helpful for plantar fasciitis are orthopedic, sports, and manual physical therapists.

Carpal Tunnel

What is it?

Your carpal tunnel is a tunnel in your wrist that is bordered on the bottom by your carpal bones (like the rocky bed of a stream) and on the top by a thick, inflexible, fibrous tissue called your flexor retinaculum. There are nine tendons and one nerve that run through your carpal tunnel, and the job of those tendons is to bend your fingers and thumb into a fist. They also help to bend your wrist forward. When there's swelling in that tunnel, either from fluid during pregnancy or from irritation of those nine tendons, the nerve running through the tunnel (the median nerve) gets compressed. That nerve provides sensation for your thumb, your pointer finger, your middle finger, and half of your ring finger on the palm side of your hand. On the back of your hand, it provides sensation to your thumb and those fingers past the last knuckle. The median nerve also operates five muscles in your hand—three muscles for your thumb and two for your first two fingers. When you have carpal tunnel syndrome, you may experience numbness or tingling in your thumb, pointer finger, middle finger, and half of your ring finger, and weakness in your thumb and first two fingers, which might make tasks like snapping a onesie or changing a diaper difficult. You may even have pain in your hand at night.

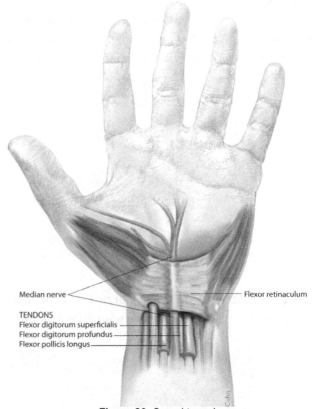

Median nerve

TENDONS
Flexor digitorum superficialis
Flexor digitorum profundus
Flexor pollicis longus

Flexor retinaculum

Figure 20. Carpal tunnel

How common is it?

Anywhere from 2–4 percent of the general population experiences carpal tunnel syndrome,[94,95] but among pregnant women that number may be as high as 70 percent.[96]

What are the risk factors?

If you have diabetes, hypothyroidism, or rheumatoid arthritis, the tissue around your tendons is often thickened, which increases the chance of compression in that tiny, rigid space. You're also at higher risk simply as a woman, and we're most likely to experience carpal tunnel syndrome during pregnancy, menopause, and if we're using birth control pills. As BMI goes up, so does our risk for carpal tunnel syndrome, and the same is true for age—we're at the highest risk after 40. Race is a risk factor too. Carpal tunnel is most common among Caucasian and Asian women. If you have a job that involves repeated fine motor activities, such as repeated grasping or holding something that's vibrating (such as operating machinery), you're more likely to irritate those tendons and experience carpal tunnel syndrome as a result.[97]

What causes it?

In pregnant women, hormonal changes result in fluid retention, and it's that fluid retention that decreases available space in the tiny, rigid carpal tunnel. Carpal tunnel syndrome can result from the decreased space due to fluid retention alone, without any tendon irritation. During breastfeeding, irritation to the tendons can become an added factor from holding the baby to breastfeed for long periods of time throughout the day and night.[96]

What's the natural course?

Carpal tunnel syndrome that starts during pregnancy usually resolves on its own as your fluid retention status returns to normal. For a small portion of women, carpal tunnel syndrome will continue so long as they're breastfeeding.[96]

What's the treatment?

For most women, carpal tunnel that started during pregnancy self-resolves without any treatment, but for those who continue to experience carpal tunnel, there are a few options. The first line of defense is to rest the tendons, and this is often achieved with a wrist brace that prevents bending the wrist forward. Occupational therapists and physical therapists can prescribe exercises and different treatments, such as hands-on manual therapy based upon individual assessments. If those non-invasive means aren't helpful, some people opt for injections of corticosteroid into their wrist, and an even smaller number of people have surgery to release the thick fibrous tissue that forms the roof of the carpal tunnel.

How can this program help?

During this program, you'll do some exercises that progressively strengthen your wrists and forearms, and that will help to prevent the development of carpal tunnel syndrome as you care for your little one.

Tweaks and tips:

If you have carpal tunnel syndrome when you start this program, you can alleviate some of the pressure through your wrists by placing a rolled hand towel under the heel of each hand during any exercise that involves placing your body weight through your hands, such as an exercise on all fours or in the plank position.

Seeking help from a physical or occupational therapist:

If you experienced carpal tunnel syndrome during pregnancy and it didn't go away after you had your baby, you may want to seek help from a physical or occupational therapist. You can find a certified hand therapist (both occupational and physical therapists can become certified as a hand therapist) at http://www.htcc.org/find-a-cht. You can use the American Physical Therapy Association website at http://www.apta.org/StateIssues/DirectAccess/ to find out if your state requires a physician referral to see a physical therapist (many states don't require a referral to see a PT, and the number is growing, but you do need a referral for an occupational therapist).

Upper Back, Neck, and Shoulder Pain

What is it?

Pain in the upper back, neck, and shoulders can take on many different forms, and among new moms, the most common include aching while sitting and while caring for the baby, stiffness with movement, and pain radiating from the neck to the shoulders and upper back. I'm grouping the three together because among new moms the cause is very often the same: mom-of-a-newborn posture.

How common is it?

Upper back, neck, and shoulder pain is very common among anyone caring for children under the age of four. In fact, it is second most common to low back pain, with 44.5 percent of parents of children under the age of four reporting pain in the upper back, neck, or shoulders.[72]

What are the risk factors?

Anyone caring for a new baby is at risk for developing this postural syndrome because of the time spent looking down at the baby, lifting the baby, carrying and rocking the baby, prolonged sitting in a posture that accommodates the baby during breastfeeding or bottle feeding but might not be optimal for you, wearing the baby in a carrier, and carrying the baby in a car seat.

What causes it?

To have good posture for a healthy neck, your ears should be positioned right over your shoulders. When your ears are far forward of your shoulders, you stretch out the muscles in the front of your neck along your spine (behind your throat). Those muscles should be helping to hold your heavy head up. Instead, the tiny muscles at the base of your skull have to pull extra hard to support your head, and in that forward position they're in a shortened position. Try jutting your chin forward and you'll see what I mean. Muscles on the front of your neck lengthen, and the muscles at the base of your skull scrunch up. They're the ones doing the work to help hold your head up.

This so-called "forward head posture" is part of a triad I'd like to call "new mom posture." The next part of "new mom posture" is a rounded upper back (think Quasimodo). As new moms, we tend to curl our upper backs forward when we're holding and feeding our babies, and over time our muscles start to get used to that position and it becomes more fixed. Holding our babies in our arms and lifting our babies over and over throughout the day causes our shoulders to naturally curve forward. The muscles that pull our arms back and rotate our shoulders out get relatively weak compared to the opposite muscles we use constantly to care for the baby. As a result, the tissue deep behind our shoulder joints (the posterior capsule) gets tight as it follows our shoulders into that rounded position, locking our shoulders down in their new forward position. All of that can result in joint and muscle pain in the neck and upper back and even disc problems that can cause radiating pain as well as shoulder pain with lifting and moving our arms above horizontal. Some women even experience headaches from the strain on the muscles at the back of the neck (those types of headaches are called "rams horn" headaches because they start at the base of the skull and then curl up around the ears to the forehead, like a ram's horns).

What's the natural course?

Postural pain tends to linger and continue to worsen until you take action to fix the posture.

What's the treatment?

The first line of defense against this type of postural problem is, of course, to fix your posture. Sometimes it's not as simple as just sitting up straight, especially when you have a baby to feed every few hours and you're exhausted. Try tweaking your nursing or baby-feeding position by using a nursing pillow, finding a pillow to put behind your low back in your favorite nursing chair, adjusting your nursing stool so that your whole back and head are supported as you feed your baby, or even lying on your side to nurse with a pillow under your head to keep your neck straight. Simple as it's not, sitting up straight *is* the first step. If you're not doing that, you're fighting a losing battle from the start.

The next steps are stretching the muscles at the base of your skull, your chest, and your shoulders, and strengthening your upper back muscles, your shoulder blade muscles, and the muscles that rotate your shoulders back. If you seek help from a physical therapist, your treatment plan will likely include personalized stretches and strengthening exercises and possibly hands-on joint mobilizations and/or manipulations, dry needling, and a variety of other treatments depending upon your physical therapist's assessment.

How can this program help?

Exercises to stretch the muscles at the base of your skull, your chest, and your shoulders, as well as strengthening exercises for your upper back muscles, your shoulder blade stabilizers, and your rotator cuff muscles, are built into this program from the beginning. "New mom posture" is so common and so problematic that it's the rule rather than the exception, and you will likely start to feel much better as you work on improving your posture.

Tweaks and tips

Here are a few extra stretches and exercises to add to your daily routine if you're having pain in your neck, upper back, or shoulders. Lying on your back on a mat or carpet, place a rolled hand towel under the base of your skull. Try to press the back of your neck towards your mat, keeping your head on your towel, until you feel the stretch as your chin tucks with the movement. Hold for 20–30 seconds. You should feel this stretch in the base of your skull and your upper back.

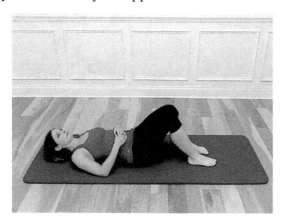 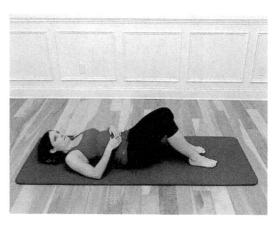

Next, remove the rolled towel from behind your head, hold your knees, and bring them toward your chest. Exhale to feel the stretch in your upper back and hold for 20–30 seconds.

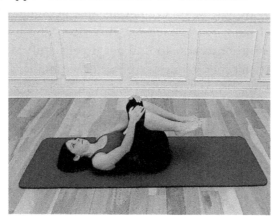

To stretch the back of your shoulders, do the sleeper stretch once or twice a day. Lying on your side with your arm out at 90 degrees and your elbow bent, very gently put pressure through your wrist as if to try to rotate your hand down to the ground. You should feel the stretch in the back of your shoulder. Hold for two sets of one minute.

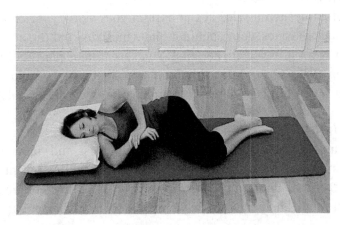

My favorite exercise for strengthening the rotator cuff is the windshield wiper. Holding a burp cloth with both hands and your elbows at your sides, forearms out straight in front of you, pull outward on the burp cloth. There shouldn't be too much give, so your arms should still be roughly parallel. Holding the tension tight and even through both hands, slowly glide your burp cloth 4 inches to the right, then 4 inches to the left. Repeat for 30 seconds.

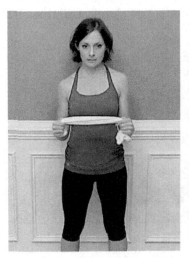 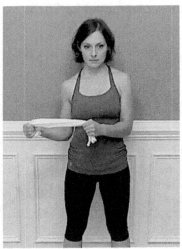 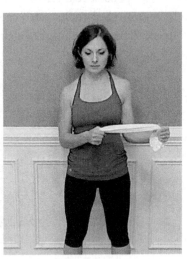

Seeking help from a physical therapist:

A physical therapist can provide you with evaluation and personalized treatment program for your neck, upper back, and/or shoulder pain. You can use the American Physical Therapy Association website at http://www.apta.org/StateIssues/DirectAccess/ to find out if your state requires a physician referral to see a physical therapist (many states don't require a referral, and the number is growing). You can use the "Find a PT" tool on their Move Forward website at http://www.moveforwardpt.com/ to find a physical therapist to help you. Particularly helpful for this type of pain are orthopedic, sports, and manual physical therapists.

"Baby wrist"

What is it?

Baby wrist is pain on the thumb side of your wrist that many moms experience while lifting their babies or doing tasks that involve pinching or grasping.[98] Its medical name is De Quervain's tenosynovitis, so yes, we'll stick to calling it Baby Wrist. There are two tendons that run through a tiny tunnel there, and in isolation they work to bring your thumb back and out to the side (tendons run from the meaty part of a muscle to attach to the bone, and the muscles attached to these tendons are the abductor pollicis longus and the extensor pollicis brevis). When those muscles work with the rest of the wrist, they help to bend your wrist back and in the direction of your thumb, exactly like you do when you're lifting your baby.

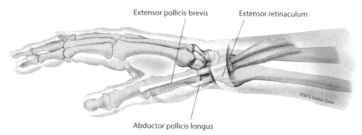

Figure 21. "Baby wrist"

How common is it?

Baby Wrist affects anywhere from 1–3 percent of the general population, and women more commonly than men.[98] Among women, it's a little more common for new mothers.

What are the risk factors?

The biggest risk factor for developing Baby Wrist is simply being a woman. If your daily life or work involves heavy use of your thumb and wrist (like picking up a baby over and over), your risk is also higher for developing baby wrist. The third major risk factor for developing Baby Wrist is being older than 40.[98]

What causes it?

When holding or lifting a baby, the typical wrist position is bent slightly forward and to the side of your pinky finger with your thumb lifting out and up. As you start to lift, you bend your whole wrist toward the side of your thumb. It turns out that puts a whole lot of tension through those two tendons involved with Baby Wrist, and that can result in swelling of the tendons and their cushioned coating. The hormonal changes of pregnancy and breastfeeding are already increasing fluid retention, so it doesn't take as much swelling to make the tiny tunnel tight enough to be painful.[99] Since the tendons are supposed to glide in their tunnel as you move your wrist, all this swelling can create a problem—every time your tendons try to glide through the tunnel, it's now too tight, so it hurts. The more swelling, the more difficult and painful it gets, creating even more swelling.

What's the natural course?

If Baby Wrist becomes chronic, over time the tendons and their cushioned coating can become thickened and more fibrous, making your wrist even more sensitive to stresses on those tendons in the future. Usually Baby Wrist will resolve on its own after your baby graduates from breastfeeding.

What's the treatment?

Most people get better from Baby Wrist with simple treatments aimed at reducing the swelling (such as ice) and simultaneously resting the wrist by using a brace that supports the thumb.[99] Sometimes it's necessary to take further steps such as a corticosteroid injection into the tiny tunnel or even surgery (though that is not common).

How can this program help?

During this program, you'll be working on strengthening your forearms and shoulders, and the stronger you are in your forearms and shoulders, the easier it will be on your wrists to lift your baby.

Tweaks and tips

If you have pain in your wrist on the thumb side, it's important to get that checked out by a health care provider, whether it's your physician or a physical therapist, especially if you can think back to one moment when your wrist started hurting, like if you fell down and landed on an outstretched hand. There are a few structures in the same area that will need immediate attention if they are the underlying cause of your wrist pain (including the scaphoid bone, which doesn't have great blood supply and does a poor job of healing on its own if you fracture it). If you do have a confirmed case of Baby Wrist and your medical care provider has given you the green light to continue exercising, keep in mind that resting those tendons is key to getting better. If it's painful even to hold a weight because of Baby Wrist, do any of the weighted exercises without weights for now. You won't be able to progress in getting better from Baby Wrist if you continue to irritate the tendons.

Seeking help from a physical therapist or occupational therapist:

If you have pain in your wrist, you should seek help from a medical care provider, and if you get the diagnosis of Baby Wrist (or De Quervain's tenosynovitis), you can seek help from a physical or occupational therapist. A certified hand therapist is the best type of physical or occupational therapist to see for Baby Wrist. You can find a certified hand therapist (both occupational and physical therapists can become certified as a hand therapist) at http://www.htcc.org/find-a-cht. You can use the American Physical Therapy Association website at http://www.apta.org/StateIssues/DirectAccess/ to find out if your state requires a physician referral to see a physical therapist (many states don't require a referral to see a PT, and the number is growing, but you do need a referral for an occupational therapist).

Quick Start Guide

You can visit my website at www.healthyquickfit.com for videos of the exercise progression, research updates, and lots of other information about gear and exercise for moms.

To access almost 10 hours of videos, including 7 hours of exclusive content, use the password **BABYFIT.**

If you just got this book and you're ready to start exercising, by all means, let's get to it! You can read the first part of this book as you go ahead with the exercises. Before getting started with our exercise routine, though, we need to cover three important topics. First, we'll go over some ground rules about safety. Second, I'll give you an overview of how to use this program. Third, we'll cover some basics, including our basic core drill (the foundation for repairing your body after pregnancy) and general rules about form for a couple other exercises.

Ground Rules

Before you start this program, it's important that your doctor clears you to exercise. If you are reading this before you have your baby, great! Put this book in your go-bag for the hospital and show the exercises to your doctor after your baby is born. After you're discharged from the hospital, it's likely your next appointment won't be for six weeks, and if you want to start exercising before then, you'll need to ask some questions. Ask if you can get started right away and if there's anything you should avoid. There may be some particulars that are specific to you, your delivery, and your situation, and your doctor can let you know if there's anything you need to avoid and for how long.

Precautions

Right after you give birth, your body is changing rapidly, and it can not only look but also *feel* unrecognizable to you, making it harder to know if something is wrong. It will be weeks or months before you feel like you "know" your body again, so I'll give you a list of some things to be on the lookout for. Stop exercising right away if you feel any of the following (items in **bold** require immediate medical attention, as in going to the Emergency Room). If you have one of the symptoms not listed in **bold**, and the symptom doesn't resolve after you stop exercising, call your doctor.

- You feel lightheaded, or become dizzy (go to the ER if it doesn't stop after a few minutes)
- **You have chest pain or feel short of breath out of proportion to your level of exertion**
- **You have a sudden, severe headache**
- You have pain in your abdomen (**if it's severe, seek medical attention immediately**)
- You have pain in the vaginal area
- **You have a sudden heavy increase in postpartum bleeding, or if you have stopped bleeding, heavy bleeding starts again**
- **You have pain or swelling in your calf**

- If you had a C-section, you should also be following your doctor's instructions to watch for signs of infection at your incision site. If you note any of these signs, you need to be seen that same day. If you are experiencing an infection, you should not be exercising until the infection has cleared AND you get clearance again from your doctor to resume.

How To Use This Program

There are 10 progressive levels for this program, and each one builds off of the level before. Start with Level 1, and only progress to the next level once you have mastered all of the exercises in the previous level and you are able to complete all of the exercises in each set without breaking mid-set to rest. Each workout is designed in the same way, with a movement prep set followed by your core drills, and then a circuit that you'll repeat three times. Circuits are great for moms of babies because workouts often happen while the baby is sleeping, and if baby should wake up after two rounds of your circuit, you have the option of completing a third round the next time you have 15 spare minutes, like the next time your baby is napping. You also have the option of being done with your workout for the day, since you've already done two good sets covering all the muscles on the schedule for that day. The last part of each workout consists of cooling down with light stretching.

On the next few pages you'll find example calendars of what a month's worth of workouts should look like. Four weeks are shown for Level 1 just to give you some pattern options, but you will likely be finished with Level 1 after the first 2 weeks. The workouts are designed to be your whole-body daily exercise routine, and the monthly calendars will show you how to pattern your circuit training (strength training) with cardio-vascular training (such as walking, running, or cycling). The sample calendars show a different pattern each week—some days you'll see a circuit plus a short cardio session, and some days you'll see a longer cardio session with no circuit. You'll also see days off on the calendar.

You can vary up your pattern each week, just like what you see on the calendar, or you can stick with a pattern that works best for you and repeat the weekly pattern. If you prefer a circuit plus a short cardio session every day, with Sunday as your rest day, you'll see that pattern as an example as the first week of the month. If you'd rather take a mid-week break and have one day of a longer cardio workout on your schedule, you'll find that pattern as the second week of the month on the calendar. If you always like to do a longer cardio workout on Saturday followed by a day off Sunday, you'll like the third and fourth weeks on the calendar—just be sure to alternate which circuit (A or B) you start your week with so that you don't end up with an imbalance over the course of a month.

If you had a C-section and/or you were on bed rest during your pregnancy, there's a special pre-program workout for you to do with your doctor's permission. Those sections are titled "C-Section" and "Bedrest." If you were on bed rest and then had a C-section, start with the C-section exercises. Once all of those exercises are easy for you and your doctor has given you the go-ahead, begin Level 1. Your doctor may give you the green light to start Level 1 if he or she sees the exercises on the list before you're cleared for exercising without any restrictions, so it is worth asking.

Otherwise, start with Level 1, no matter how fit you are. For the first 6 weeks, you will still be healing. The workouts in Levels 1 to 3 are designed to protect your body during the healing phase, so you should progress no faster than 1 level every 2 weeks for the first 3 levels. Two weeks is also the amount of time it takes to re-establish movement patterns, and that is very important during the first 3 levels of this program. After the first 3 levels, you can progress as quickly as 1 level per week, though it may take longer. Everyone will progress at a different rate, and your rate may vary by levels. Some levels may be easy after a week or 2, and other levels may take you a month or 2 to master. For each level you will need to go slowly at first and take breaks during sets.

If you're exercising with the video, keep the video rolling as you take your breaks so that as you get stronger, you'll be able to increase your repetitions to eventually keep up with me and complete the number of repetitions I'm doing. If an exercise feels too easy the first time you do it, slow down and do the exercise in a slow, controlled way. If you're exercising with the video, don't go any faster than me—that way you won't short-change yourself on exercises that are most beneficial when done in a slow, controlled way.

Your cardio progressions are in Appendices A, B, and C. Appendix A is your walk progression, Appendix B contains your cycling progression and workouts, and Appendix C includes a "Ready to Run?" core test (the Sahrmann core test), a solo running progression, and a stroller running progression. When you feel you may be ready to start running, test your core with the Sahrmann core test in Appendix C. Your physician will likely clear you to run based solely upon your reproductive tissue healing time. Your musculoskeletal tissue will take much longer to heal. Restrengthening and learning movement patterns takes longer than simple tissue healing; you'll be detraining your pregnancy patterns of movement and retraining your body to fire the right muscles in the right order to function. If you try to run before your musculoskeletal system is ready, particularly your core, you're at best going to shortchange your performance, and at worst you'll get injured. When you feel ready and you pass the Sahrmann core test in Appendix C to be at least a Level 3 on her scale, you're ready to start a run progression.

Vaginal Tearing or Episiotomy During Delivery

If you had any tearing during a vaginal delivery, it's important to discuss the extent of that tearing with your doctor or midwife before starting an exercise program or starting Kegel exercises (contracting your pelvic floor muscles). Your doctor or midwife may not discuss this with you as standard discharge instructions unless you ask, so the question you should be asking is, "When can I start doing pelvic floor or Kegel exercises?"

Vaginal tearing is classified into four degrees of laceration based upon the extent of the injury:

➢ **First degree:** Involves just the skin and tissue just beneath the skin, but no muscles.
➢ **Second degree:** Involves everything in a first degree injury plus some of the muscles of your pelvic floor, including your levator ani muscle group, but the anal sphincter muscles are not involved.
➢ **Third degree:** Involves everything in a second degree injury plus your anal sphincter muscles.
➢ **Fourth degree:** Involves everything in a third degree plus the rectal mucosa (the injury has gone all the way through to your rectum).

If you had an episiotomy, that is automatically at least a second degree laceration. Any time the pelvic floor muscles are injured (second to fourth degree lacerations) and need to be sutured, it's important to rest those muscles long enough to heal. Even with a first degree laceration, you will likely need to take time before beginning Kegels to allow the sutures to hold. Only your obstetrician will be able to tell you how long that should take, based upon the number, type, and location of sutures that you needed. Usually, although your situation may be different, so again, talk to your obstetrician, that means one week before you can start Kegels for first degree, two weeks for third degree, and three+ weeks for third and fourth degree lacerations.

For this program, that means your initial core drill may just be a wide rib breath + a belly button pull with NO pelvic floor contraction for the first week or more, depending on your obstetrician's answer.

Sample Weekly Calendars for Level 1

Stay at Level 1 for at least two weeks

During Level 1, a week might look like:

Monday	Tuesday	Wednesday	Thursday	Friday	Saturday	Sunday
Circuit A + 5–15 min. Cardio	Circuit B + 5–15 min. Cardio	Circuit A + 5–15 min. Cardio	Circuit B + 5–15 min. Cardio	Circuit A + 5–15 min. Cardio	Circuit B + 5–15 min. Cardio	Day Off

Or, if you would like to have two days of longer cardio workouts:

Monday	Tuesday	Wednesday	Thursday	Friday	Saturday	Sunday
Circuit A + 5–15 min. Cardio	Circuit B + 5–15 min. Cardio	10–20 min. Cardio	Day Off	10–20 min. Cardio	Circuit A + 5–15 min. Cardio	Circuit B + 5–15 min. Cardio

Or, if you would like to do one day of a longer cardio workout per week, two weeks might look like:

Monday	Tuesday	Wednesday	Thursday	Friday	Saturday	Sunday
Circuit A + 5–15 min. Cardio	Circuit B + 5–15 min. Cardio	Circuit A + 5–15 min. Cardio	Circuit B + 5–15 min. Cardio	Circuit A + 5–15 min. Cardio	10–20 min. Cardio	Day Off
Circuit B + 5–15 min. Cardio	Circuit A + 5–15 min. Cardio	Circuit B + 5–15 min. Cardio	Circuit A + 5–15 min. Cardio	Circuit B + 5–15 min. Cardio	10–20 min. Cardio	Day Off

CARDIO= ANY OF THE FOLLOWING

Walking

Start out with a stroll (or waddle) around the block with your baby in the stroller. Day one, just aims for 5 minutes, and over the next week or two try to go just a little farther. Speed is of no concern during these first few weeks—your body is in healing mode, so take it easy.

Run Progression

Your body won't be ready to start running during Level 1. You can start testing your core (see the Sahrmann core test, Appendix C) once you reach Level 3, but you're more likely to be ready during Level 4 or later.

Biking, Elliptical, and More

Whatever your home or gym cardio preference, whether it's the spin bike, rower, or elliptical, start out slow for the first few weeks, and gradually add intensity first, then duration second to progress in increments.

Sample Weekly Calendars for Levels 2 and Beyond

Stay at Levels 2–3 for at least two weeks and Levels 4–10 for at least one week per level

During Levels 2 and beyond, a week might look like:

Monday	Tuesday	Wednesday	Thursday	Friday	Saturday	Sunday
Circuit A + 20–30 min. Cardio	Circuit B + 20–30 min. Cardio	Circuit A + 20–30 min. Cardio	Circuit B + 20–30 min. Cardio	Circuit A + 20–30 min. Cardio	Circuit B + 20–30 min. Cardio	Day Off

Or, if you would like to have two days of longer cardio workouts:

Monday	Tuesday	Wednesday	Thursday	Friday	Saturday	Sunday
Circuit A + 20–30 min. Cardio	Circuit B + 20–30 min. Cardio	30–60 min. Cardio	Day Off	30–60 min. Cardio	Circuit A + 20–30 min. Cardio	Circuit B + 20–30 min. Cardio

Or, if you would like to do one day of a longer cardio workout per week, two weeks might look like:

Monday	Tuesday	Wednesday	Thursday	Friday	Saturday	Sunday
Circuit A + 20–30 min. Cardio	Circuit B + 20–30 min. Cardio	Circuit A + 20–30 min. Cardio	Circuit B + 20–30 min. Cardio	Circuit A + 20–30 min. Cardio	30–60 min. Cardio	Day Off
Monday	**Tuesday**	**Wednesday**	**Thursday**	**Friday**	**Saturday**	**Sunday**
Circuit B + 20–30 min. Cardio	Circuit A + 20–30 min. Cardio	Circuit B + 20–30 min. Cardio	Circuit A + 20–30 min. Cardio	Circuit B + 20–30 min. Cardio	30–60 min. Cardio	Day Off

CARDIO= ANY OF THE FOLLOWING

Walking

Simple and basic, a brisk walk with the stroller is something you and your baby can enjoy together. Start out easy, and when you're ready to work up a sweat shoot for a 15-minute per mile or faster pace.

Run Progression

Once your doctor clears you and you're able to pass the core strength test in Appendix C (Level 3 or later), you can start the run progression. Ask your pediatrician if your little one is ready for a spin in the jogging stroller. Run progressions are in Appendix C.

Biking, Elliptical, and More

You can find cycling workouts in Appendix B, and if you'd like, you can use these workouts for the elliptical too. As you progress, gradually add intensity first, then duration second to progress in increments.

The Basics

Before we get started with our workouts, we need to learn some basic skills that you'll use throughout the program. In this section, we're going to cover your core drill, posture, and squatting and lunging form. These skills are fundamental to your recovery. Mastering these skills before you get started will ensure you get the most out of your workouts, speed up your recovery process, and prevent injury.

Basic Core Drill

The core drill is made up of three movements: a wide rib breath, a pelvic floor contraction, and a transversus abdominis contraction. From here on out we'll call the transversus abdominis contraction your belly button pull. First practice these three movements independently and then put them together for a core drill. Before you start practicing these movements, especially if you had a C-section, episiotomy, or second-degree or greater tearing with a vaginal birth, be absolutely sure to get the go-ahead form your doctor.

Wide Rib Breath

Place your hands on your rib cage and take a deep breath through your nose. As you breathe in, imagine filling your rib cage with air, and your hands should move apart as you inhale. This type of breathing will maximize your diaphragm's activation, which will in turn act as a springboard for an optimal pelvic floor contraction.

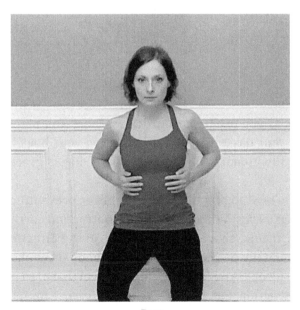

Rest

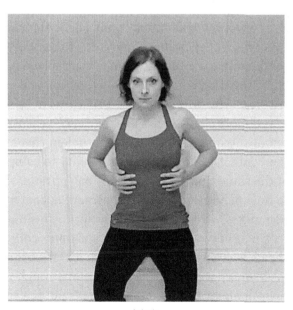

Inhale

Some common mistakes people make with taking a wide rib breath are taking a deep breath too high or taking a belly breath.

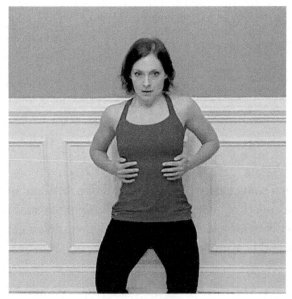

Too High

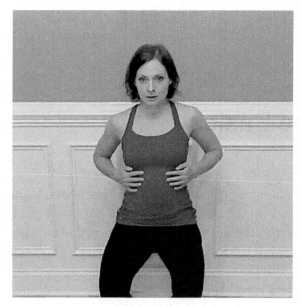

Belly Breath

Pelvic Floor Contraction (Kegel)

The second movement for your core drill is the pelvic floor contraction. Your pelvic floor is like a sling that sits at the base of your pelvis. A healthy pelvic floor helps you stay continent by preventing urine leaks or fecal accidents, helps with sexual function, and of course plays an important role and takes a beating during pregnancy and labor, even if you have a C-section. A healthy pelvic floor also serves as an absolutely integral member of your core team that's made up of your diaphragm, your deepest abdominal muscle (your transversus abdominis), your pelvic floor muscles, and your deepest back muscles. If you work on your abdominal core muscles alone, your core will not be able to function correctly as you function and exercise. At best, you will struggle to reach your athletic

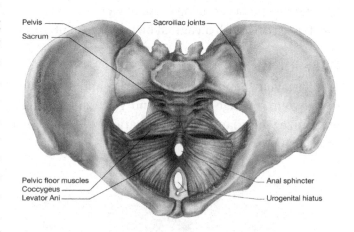

Pelvic floor musculature

goals, and more likely you will experience repeated injuries as you progress your fitness level. You may also worsen or introduce a pelvic floor problem that's affecting your day-to-day life by affecting your bowel and bladder control, sexual function, or ability to complete daily functional tasks such as lifting a bag of groceries and at the same time hold your baby on your hip.

To do a pelvic floor muscle contraction, contract as if you're stopping the flow of urine or preventing the passage of gas without squeezing your buttocks or your ab muscles. When you do the contraction correctly, the area just between your vagina and anus, called your perineum, should move upward, in the direction of your head, ever so slightly. You can check this contraction manually on the outside of your body through your clothes if you're wearing thin clothing or through your underwear. If you bear down, you'll feel that area move downward, towards your feet, and that's not the correct contraction, but it can serve as a reference for feeling for the right contraction. You can also check this contraction using a mirror. Many women are uncomfortable looking at their nether-region right after having a baby, but it won't be as bad as you imagine. If you opt to check this way, lie on your back with a pillow under your hips and hold a mirror so that you can see your perineum clearly. When you do the contraction correctly, you should see your perineum or anus move inwards towards your body, also described as upward towards your head. If you're not sure that you're getting this contraction right, it's best to see a physical therapist or obstetrician who can check this contraction for you. There are a few ways practitioners can check, including manually or with a diagnostic ultrasound machine that's used to look at muscles for biofeedback (the sound head is placed on your lower belly).

There is some old information out there that advises checking the contraction by stopping the flow of urine mid-stream, but research tells us nowadays that not only can that cause more problems if you make a habit of checking that way, but you *can* stop the flow of urine with an incorrect contraction anyway. Research has shown that the best verbal cue for contracting your pelvic floor muscles is to think of stopping the passage of gas without squeezing your buttocks, and an easy way to self check is to do a manual check through your clothing or a visual check with a mirror while lying down.[86]

You'll need to do some of these contractions in *addition* to your workout program after pregnancy to awaken and retrain those muscles as a concentrated effort. Start out practicing on your back or side, and gradually progress to doing them standing or sitting, doing a 3 second hold, then a 6 second rest, for 10–15 reps 3 times a day. That sounds like a lot, but it works out to be a maximum 2 minute 15 second exercise 3 times daily. That's 6 minutes and 45 seconds a day. The worst time to do these contractions is at the very end of the day when you're going to sleep because you're tired, those muscles are tired, and you're just not going to get the highest quality contractions.

Belly Button Pull

The third movement for your core drill is your transversus abdominis contraction, or your belly button pull. To do that contraction, lie on your back and get your spine into a neutral position. Your lower back shouldn't be pushed down into your mat so that you're tilting your pelvis back, and you don't want to arch it all the way in the other direction. Rock your pelvis forward and back until you find a comfortable spot somewhere in the middle. From that position, use your muscles to pull your belly button slowly down towards your spine. You can check your contraction with your hands by placing your fingers on your front hip bones, then moving in one inch. At that location you should feel a nice soft spot when your muscles are relaxed.

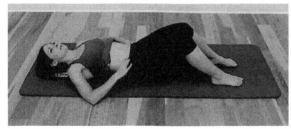
Rest

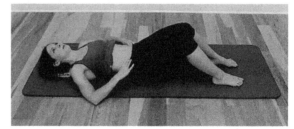
Belly Button Pull

If you contract really hard like you're doing a crunch, you'll feel a rapid jerky movement and your muscles pushing forward. A correct contraction will feel like a gradual tension rising under your fingers. Imagine a string attached to the back of your belly button. Use your muscles to pull that string and your belly button slightly back towards your spine. It's important that you're not bearing down like you're doing a crunch to do this movement, nor are you sucking in to hollow out your belly.

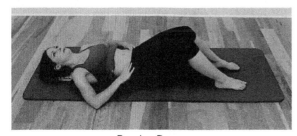
Bearing Down

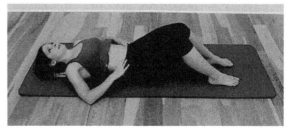
Sucking In

This should be a nice controlled movement, just drawing your belly button slowly back towards your spine. Again, if you're not sure if you're getting this contraction correct, have your physical therapist or doctor check it before you get started with the program – this core drill is essential to your success.

Putting the Pieces Together

Putting the pieces together for your core drill, we're going to load our springboard with a deep, wide rib breath in, and at the bottom of your exhale as you breathe out, do a pelvic floor contraction. Keep that pelvic floor contraction and move right into your belly button pull. The next time you breathe in again, relax your pelvic floor and your abdominal muscles completely. Sometimes relaxing is the hardest part. Practice the pieces of this core drill separately, then put them together and make sure before you start the program you're comfortable doing a good core drill. This will be the foundation of your recovery.

Posture

When you're pregnant, some women accommodate for the extra load by arching their back more and moving their upper body forward, and some women move the opposite way by gliding back.

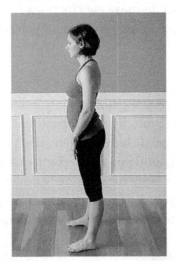 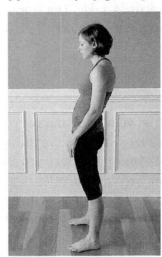

Pregnant Posture

After you have the baby, it's common to drift into that pregnancy posture again because your nerves and muscles have gotten so used to working in that posture, and now that you've had the baby, you're still carrying an extra load, but you're carrying it in your arms instead of your belly. In your weakened, post-delivery state, your body will reinforce those pregnancy patterns to try to help you accommodate the growing load in your arms. It takes a bit of diligence, but you can get your posture back into a healthy position that will improve your recovery and prevent injuries. Throughout the day and during your workouts, start to routinely check your posture. Place your rib cage right over your pelvis, drop your shoulders down away from your ears, and move your head back so that your ears are directly over your shoulders.

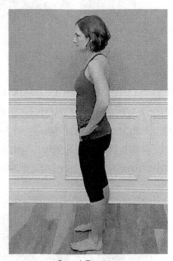

Good Posture

Squatting

The most common mistakes women make when squatting are leading with our knees, letting our knees roll in, and putting the weight through our toes.

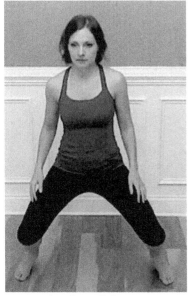 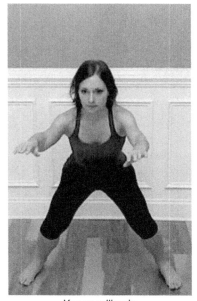 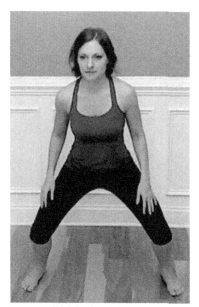

Leading with knees   Knees rolling in   Weight through toes

To squat, the first movement should be gliding your hips back, rather than bending your knees. That hip glide will guide your knees into the bend for your squat. Practice this daily starting now at your kitchen counter so that when we start doing squats as part of the program, you'll be ready. Hips back, then lower down, with your weight through your heels. Do 20–30 mini-squats per day, just working on getting your hips back and going down a few inches into a squat.

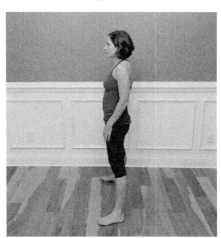 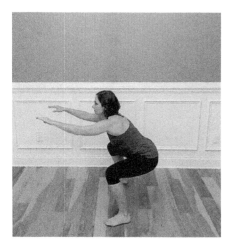

When you start to do the squats for the workouts, you'll be going lower and lower as you get better, and the rule with squatting is to keep your knees behind your toes. You can check by looking at your toes. If your knees block the view of your toes, you're moving your knees too far forward and you need to put your weight more through your heels. For some people, this means doing mini squats or squats holding on to a counter for a long time before they can break horizontal without their knees going forward of their toes. You may need to start out watching in a mirror to make sure your knees aren't collapsing inward when you squat.

Lunges

When you lunge, you need to keep your back straight and, again, keep your knees behind your toes. Don't start lunging until you reach that part of the program, but here's a sample of what a correct lunge looks like so that you know now.

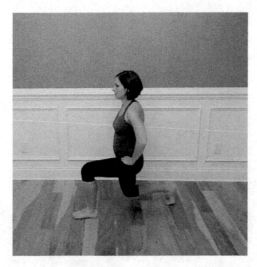

Once you master your core drill basics and you're working on your posture and counter mini-squats throughout the day, you're ready to start Level 1!

Bed Rest

During Bed Rest

If you are on bed rest now and reading this book before you give birth, great! Your doctor *may* allow you to do some exercises. Before doing any exercises, make sure you have very clear approval from your obstetrician. Show the following chart to your obstetrician and have him or her approve each exercise you are allowed to do. With your doctor's approval, you can make a mini-circuit out of those approved exercises and repeat the sequence of approved exercises one to three times daily. Also, make sure you've read the "Ground Rules" before starting.

During Bed Rest Mini-Workout

Do only the exercises your obstetrician approves of, in order, one to three times daily. If you feel any pain or have any bleeding, loss of fluid, lightheadedness, dizziness, decreased fetal movement, onset of contractions, or pain, stop the exercises and immediately notify your obstetrician.

Do this workout one to three times daily

You Will Need:
- 5–9 Minutes
- A mat and a chair, or just your bed
- Water

When you sit up from lying down, roll to your side first instead of sitting straight up. Instead of struggling to sit straight up, roll onto your side, move your legs to the edge, and swing your legs down as you push your torso up with your arms.

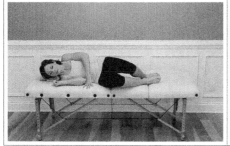 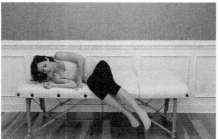 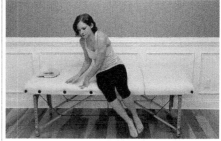

Doctor Approval?	Circuit			
Yes No	**Flys** **20 reps**	• Start with arms straight out, palms together • As you inhale, move your arms all the way out to the side, opening your chest • Breathe out to bring your arms back • Keep your arms up for the next exercise		
Yes No	**Scaption** **20 reps**	• Move your arms in to about a 45 degree angle • Lift straight up towards the ceiling, thumbs up • Come back down past horizontal		
Yes No	**Knee Extension** **20 per side**	• Straighten your knee • At the top, really tighten your thigh muscle		
Stand up tall and hold onto something for balance. Do 20 marches in place, taking good, full breaths. If you feel lightheaded or dizzy, sit back down, take a few deep breaths, and stand up a little slower to try again. If you do need to try again, just stand and take a few deep breaths at first.				
Yes No	**Mini-Calf Raise** **20 reps**	• Come up onto your toes with your heels lifting about one inch off the ground		

Doctor Approval?	Circuit		
Yes No	**Counter Squats** **20 reps**	• Hold on to the kitchen counter for support • Glide your hips back first to introduce the bend in your knees • Start with a very shallow squat, and go deeper only as you get stronger	
Yes No	**Tush Sway** **20 per side**	• Stand with feet more than shoulder width apart • Rock your weight side to side using your outer hip muscles to push • Come up onto your toes as you push off of each side	
Yes No	**Mini-Glute Pump** **10 per side**	• Stand on one leg • With the other knee bent, pump your foot straight back to feel your glute working	

		Cool Down	
Yes

No | **Calf Stretch**

15 sec. per side | • Stand stagger-step, and hold on for balance
• Bend your front knee
• Keep your back heel on the ground
• Feel the stretch in your calf | |
| Yes

No | **Thigh + Low Calf Stretch**

15 sec. per side | • Keep the stagger-step position
• Bend your back knee
• Release your heel from the floor
• Tuck your butt under
• Feel the stretch in the front of your hip and thigh and in your low calf | |
| Yes

No | **Hamstring Stretch**

15 sec. per side | • Prop your heel forward
• Pull your hips back
• Keep the small of your back arched
• Feel the stretch in the back of your thigh | |

After Bed Rest

If you were on bed rest and had a vaginal delivery, the following circuit is your starting point for exercise. Make sure you've read the "Ground Rules" and mastered "The Basics" before starting. Do this mini-exercise routine daily along with your walking routine until you're able to do all of the exercises correctly and you can do all of the reps listed. Once this routine is fairly easy for you, progress to Level 1 of the program.

Getting up again

After spending some time confined to bed rest, you may feel ready to jump out of bed and hit your new exercise routine hard, but there are lots of reasons to take it slow at first. You may experience a sudden drop in blood pressure when you change positions, like going from lying down to sitting up or sitting up to standing, and that drop in blood pressure can make you feel lightheaded, dizzy, or faint, and it can even cause you to fall down. This symptom is called postural hypotension, and it's very common after spending some time on bed rest.

After you've been on bed rest, your body's natural ability to regulate your blood pressure is impaired. Normally, when you move into an upright position and gravity moves your blood down towards your feet, your body responds by constricting your blood vessels to help move the blood back up towards your head. After prolonged bed rest, your blood vessels are out of practice, and this response is delayed. It's important to change positions slowly at first to avoid falling down and to get your blood vessels back in shape and in good working order again.

A landmark study published in 2000 showed that 3 weeks of bed rest took a greater toll on 5 healthy, 20-year-old men than did 30 years of aging. In 1966, a group of researchers placed 5 healthy young men on bed rest for 3 weeks and measured the immediate effects on their bodies. The men were released to recover and live normal lives. Thirty years later, the same 5 men returned to the researchers, who took the same measurements again, this time looking for the effects of 30 years of aging. As it turned out, the 3 weeks of bed rest had a greater negative impact on the men's cardiovascular systems (particularly their bodies' ability to transport oxygen to their muscles and their physical work capacity) than 30 years of aging.[100] Getting up again after being on bed rest is not as simple as you may hope. These negative effects after bed rest are temporary, but it's important to understand why getting moving again may seem so difficult at first. Don't get frustrated. Take it slow, listen to your body (and your doctor), and you'll recover just fine.

Post Bed Rest Mini-Workout

Do this workout if your doctor approves of these exercises until you can do all of the exercises correctly and with ease. At that point, you can begin Level 1.

Do this workout one to three times daily

You Will Need:
- 9 Minutes
- A mat and a chair, or just your bed
- Water

Core Drill Exercise		
Basic Core Drill **10 reps**	• Wide rib breath in • Kegel on exhale • Move right into belly button pull • Relax Kegel and belly button pull to breathe in again	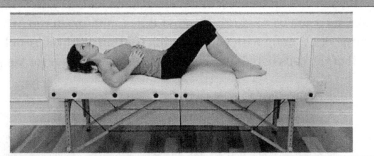

When you sit up from lying down, roll to your side first instead of sitting straight up. Instead of struggling to sit straight up, roll onto your side, move your legs to the edge, and swing your legs down as you push your torso up with your arms.

Circuit		
Flys **20 reps**	• Start with arms straight out, palms together • As you inhale, move your arms all the way out to the side, opening your chest • Breathe out to bring your arms back • Keep your arms up for the next exercise	
Scaption **20 reps**	• Move your arms in to about a 45 degree angle • Lift straight up towards the ceiling, thumbs up • Come back down past horizontal	
Quad Kicks **20 per side**	• With toes pointed, straighten your knee • Tap your toes on the mat/floor	

Stand up tall and hold onto something for balance. Do 20 marches in place, taking good full breaths. If you feel lightheaded or dizzy, sit back down, take a few deep breaths, and stand up a little slower to try again. If you do need to try again, just stand and take a few deep breaths at first.

Mini-Calf Raise **20 reps**	Come up onto your toes with your heels lifting about one inch off the ground		
Counter Squats **20 reps**	• Hold on to the kitchen counter for support • Glide your hips back first to introduce the bend in your knees • Start with a very shallow squat, and go deeper only as you get stronger		
Tush Sway **20 per side**	• Stand with feet more than shoulder width apart • Rock your weight side to side using your outer hip muscles to push • Come up onto your toes as you push off of each side		
Mini-Glute Pump **10 per side**	• Stand on one leg • With the other knee bent, pump your foot straight back to feel your glute working		

Calf Stretch **15 sec. per side**	• Stand stagger-step, and hold on for balance • Bend your front knee • Keep your back heel on the ground • Feel the stretch in your calf	
Thigh + Low Calf Stretch **15 sec. per side**	• Keep the stagger-step position • Bend your back knee • Release your heel from the floor • Tuck your butt under • Feel the stretch in the front of your hip and thigh and in your low calf	
Hamstring Stretch **15 sec. per side**	• Prop your heel forward • Pull your hips back • Keep the small of your back arched • Feel the stretch in the back of your thigh	

C-Section

If you had a C-section, whether or not you were on bed rest, the following circuit is your starting point for exercise, only with your doctor's approval. Ask your doctor for approval of these exercises before starting if he or she had to cut through any muscle tissue during the C-section, or if there is any reason to be extra cautious during your recovery. Make sure you've read the "Ground Rules" and "The Basics" before starting. Do this mini-exercise routine daily along with your walking routine until you're able to do all of the exercises correctly and you can do all of the exercises without taking breaks mid-set. Once this routine is fairly easy for you and your doctor clears you for all exercises, including transversus abdominis or abdominal muscle work, progress to Level 1 of the program. For this routine you will need a mat and a chair or just a bed.

C-sections: They're not all the same

There are two main types of initial C-section incisions through your skin: horizontal or vertical. Your surgery, though it may have seemed quick, involved incisions through many different layers of tissue to get to (and then through) your uterus. The healing incision you see on your skin may or may not match the incisions on each deeper layer, depending upon the technique necessary for your particular situation.[13]

For most C-sections, your doctor will make a low incision horizontally, and each layer beneath the skin will follow similar horizontal lines. During this type of C-section, the doctor is able to avoid cutting any of the actual muscle tissue. Instead, the incisions are through a type of tissue called fascia, which connects your abdominal tissue together and to bone.[13] Fascia is thick, fibrous tissue. Even though fascia doesn't contract, you will put tension on the healing incisions in your fascia by contracting certain abdominal muscles, since the muscles attach to the fascia. For that reason, you should avoid abdominal muscle work until the doctor who performed your C-section clears you to start. Some doctors may approve certain kinds of gentle core activation, and others may advise avoiding abdominal muscle work altogether; that depends on your particular surgery.

Vertical incisions also typically involve incisions through fascia and not actual muscle tissue, but because of the direction of pull for certain abdominal muscles, abdominal muscle activation can put more tension on this type of incision, and you'll have to be a little more cautious. Even with a horizontal incision that may appear simple from the outside, there is a chance that the surgeon had to cut through, and then reattach, the tendons of some of the muscles at the attachment to the bone.[13] If you had this type of C-section, your doctor will likely be much more strict about avoiding certain activities during the healing process. If you know someone with a C-section incision that appears the same as yours on the skin, but her advice to resume exercising is much more liberal than yours, don't assume your doctor is just being too cautious.

Remember, the incision on the skin doesn't tell the whole story. Since many forms of exercise recruit your abdominal muscles involuntarily, it's important to discuss the specifics of any exercise program with your doctor before starting.

Post C-Section Mini-Workout

Do this workout if your doctor approves of these exercises until your doctor gives the go-ahead for all exercises. At that point, you can begin Level 1.

Do this workout one to three times daily

You will need:
- 9 Minutes
- A mat and a chair, or just your bed
- Water

Core Drill Exercise		
Wide Rib Breath + Pelvic Floor Contraction **10 reps**	• Wide rib breath in • Kegel on exhale* • Relax Kegel to breathe in again	

* If your doctor has cleared you to work on your transversus abdominis or your core, add the belly button pull maneuver after your pelvic floor contraction, making this exercise a full core drill: deep wide rib breath, pelvic floor contraction, then belly button pull. Relax to inhale, contract at the bottom of your exhale.

When you sit up from lying down, roll to your side first instead of sitting straight up. Instead of struggling to sit straight up, roll onto your side, move your legs to the edge, and swing your legs down as you push your torso up with your arms.

Circuit		
Flys **20 reps**	• Start with arms straight out, palms together • As you inhale, move your arms all the way out to the side, opening your chest • Breathe out to bring your arms back • Keep your arms up for the next exercise	
Scaption **20 reps**	• Move your arms in to about a 45 degree angle • Lift straight up towards the ceiling, thumbs up • Come back down past horizontal	

86

Knee Extension **20 per side**	• Straighten your knee • At the top, really tighten your thigh muscle	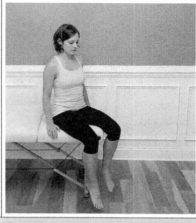	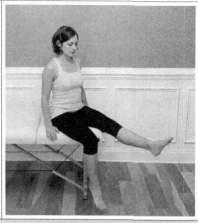

Stand up tall and hold onto something for balance. Do 20 marches in place, taking good, full breaths. If you feel lightheaded or dizzy, sit back down, take a few deep breaths, and stand up a little slower to try again. If you do need to try again, just stand and take a few deep breaths at first.

Mini-Calf Raise **20 reps**	• Come up onto your toes with your heels lifting about one inch off the ground	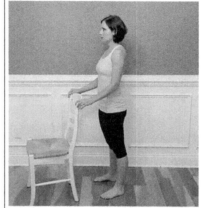	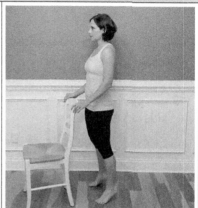
Counter Squats **20 reps**	• Hold on to the kitchen counter for support • Glide your hips back first to introduce the bend in your knees • Start with a very shallow squat, and go deeper only as you get stronger	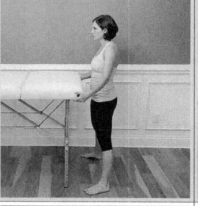	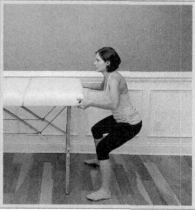
Tush Sway **20 per side**	• Stand with feet more than shoulder width apart • Rock your weight side to side using your outer hip muscles to push • Come up onto your toes as you push off of each side	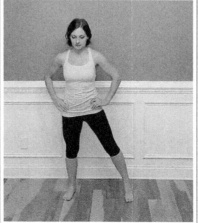	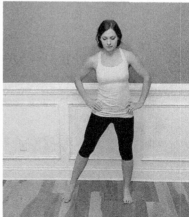

Mini-Glute Pump **10 per side**	• Stand on one leg • With the other knee bent, pump your foot straight back to feel your glute working		

Cool Down

Calf Stretch **15 sec. per side**	• Stand stagger-step, and hold on for balance • Bend your front knee • Keep your back heel on the ground • Feel the stretch in your calf	
Thigh + Low Calf Stretch **15 sec. per side**	• Keep the stagger-step position • Bend your back knee • Release your heel from the floor • Tuck your butt under • Feel the stretch in the front of your hip and thigh and in your low calf	
Hamstring Stretch **15 sec. per side**	• Prop your heel forward • Pull your hips back • Keep the small of your back arched • Feel the stretch in the back of your thigh	

Circuit Workouts

Uncomplicated Vaginal Delivery

If you had an uncomplicated vaginal delivery, you can begin with Level 1, so long as your doctor approves of you starting this exercise program. Be sure you've read the "Ground Rules" and that you've mastered "The Basics" before getting started.

Complicated Delivery (Including Multiples)

If you had a complicated delivery, be sure you show these exercises to your doctor before getting started. You'll need your doctor's approval for each exercise to be safe. If you were on bed rest, start with the Bed Rest section first, and if you had a C-section, start with the C-section first. You will need to progress to Level 1 with your doctor's approval.

Level 1

Circuit A

Before starting Level 1, you should have mastered the exercises titled "The Basics." If not, go back and review and master those basic exercises. They are fundamental to your success with this entire program.

Alternate Circuit A one day and Circuit B the next day for a 21 minute workout 4–6 times a week.

You Will Need:

- 21 Minutes
- A mat
- Water
- A towel
- Your kitchen counter

Core Drill Exercises: Repeat core drill exercises for a total of 2 rounds of each exercise		
Basic Core Drill **5 reps**	• Wide rib breath in • Kegel on exhale • Move right into belly button pull • Relax your pelvic floor and abdominal muscles to breathe in again	
Core Drill Exercise— Slow March **5 per side**	• Inhale and exhale between each movement • On each exhale, do a core drill (Kegel, then belly button pull) • On each inhale, relax core (abdominal muscles and Kegel) • During: • 1st Exhale and core drill: Lift your heel and hold it up • 2nd Exhale and core drill: Lift your whole foot 1 inch off the floor • 3rd Exhale and core drill: Lower your foot • Continue steps 1–3 to alternate sides for 5 reps per side	

Circuit: Do all 3 exercises in order, and repeat 2 more times for a total of 3 rounds			
Panini Press **20 per side**	• Start with your body in an "L" shape • Lift your top leg as a whole • Lower to repeat 20 times		
Clamshells **20 per side**	• Start with your body in fetal position • Open your knees, keeping your feet together like a clamshell • Lower to repeat 20 times		
Counter Squats **20 per side**	• Hold on to your kitchen counter/door frame • Feet more than shoulder width apart • Weight through heels • Slide hips back • Allow knees to bend • Keep knees behind toes • Stand back up, driving through heels		
STOP: Take a break to get some water between rounds. Repeat the circuit for 2 more rounds.			

Light Stretching		
Calf Stretch **15 sec. per side**	• Stand stagger-step, and hold on for balance • Bend your front knee • Keep your back heel on the ground • Feel the stretch in your calf	
Thigh + Low Calf Stretch **15 sec. per side**	• Keep the stagger-step position • Bend your back knee • Release your heel from the floor • Tuck your butt under • Feel the stretch in the front of your hip and thigh and in your low calf	
Hamstring Stretch **15 sec. per side**	• Prop your heel forward • Pull your hips back • Keep the small of your back arched • Feel the stretch in the back of your thigh	
Chin Tuck **10 reps**	• Pull your head straight back • Add a little extra pressure with your hand • Feel the stretch at the base of your skull	
Cat Stretch **20–30 sec. per side**	• Reach for the right side of the mat • Curve your body into a "C" as you sit back • Feel the stretch on your left side and lower back • Switch sides and repeat	

Level 1

Circuit B

Before starting Level 1, you should have mastered the exercises titled "The Basics." If not, go back and review and master those basic exercises. They are fundamental to your success with this entire program.

Alternate Circuit A one day and Circuit B the next day for a 21 minute workout 4–6 times a week.

You Will Need:
- 21 Minutes
- A mat
- Water
- A towel
- A chair

Core Drill Exercises: Repeat core drill exercises for a total of 2 rounds of each exercise		
Basic Core Drill **5 reps**	• Wide rib breath in • Kegel on exhale • Move right into belly button pull • Relax your pelvic floor and abdominal muscles to breathe in again	
Core Drill Exercise— Slow March **5 per side**	• Inhale and exhale between each movement • On each exhale, do a core drill (Kegel, then belly button pull) • On each inhale, relax core (abdominal muscles and Kegel) • During: • 1st Exhale and core drill: Lift your heel and hold it up • 2nd Exhale and core drill: Lift your whole foot 1 inch off the floor • 3rd Exhale and core drill: Lower your foot • Continue steps 1–3 to alternate sides for 5 reps per side	

Circuit: Do all 3 exercises in order, and repeat 2 more times for a total of 3 rounds			
All Fours Beginner Glute Lifts **15 per side**	• Start out on all fours • Keeping your knee bent, bring your leg halfway up, lifting your foot towards the ceiling		
Flys **20 reps**	• Start with arms straight out, palms together • As you inhale, move your arms all the way out to the side, opening your chest • Breathe out to bring your arms back • Keep your arms up for the next exercise		
Scaption **20 reps**	• Move your arms in to about a 45 degree angle • Lift straight up towards the ceiling, thumbs up • Come back down past horizontal		
STOP: Take a break to get some water between rounds. Repeat the circuit for 2 more rounds.			

Light Stretching

Calf Stretch **15 sec. per side**	• Stand stagger-step, and hold on for balance • Bend your front knee • Keep your back heel on the ground • Feel the stretch in your calf	
Thigh + Low Calf Stretch **15 sec. per side**	• Keep the stagger-step position • Bend your back knee • Release your heel from the floor • Tuck your butt under • Feel the stretch in the front of your hip and thigh and in your low calf	
Hamstring Stretch **15 sec. per side**	• Prop your heel forward • Pull your hips back • Keep the small of your back arched • Feel the stretch in the back of your thigh	
Chin Tuck **10 reps**	• Pull your head straight back • Add a little extra pressure with your hand • Feel the stretch at the base of your skull	
Cat Stretch **20–30 sec. per side**	• Reach for the right side of the mat • Curve your body into a "C" as you sit back • Feel the stretch on your left side and lower back • Switch sides and repeat	

Level 2

Circuit A

Before starting Level 2, you should have mastered all of the exercises from Level 1. If not, continue Level 1 until you can do all of the exercises in Level 1 correctly and without taking mid-set breaks.

Alternate Circuit A one day and Circuit B the next day for an 18–24 minute workout 4–6 times a week.

You Will Need:

- 18 Minutes
- A mat
- Water
- A towel
- A pillow (a nursing pillow works great)

Core Drill Exercises: Repeat core drill exercises for a total of 2 rounds of each exercise		

Core Drill Exercise— Supine March
 	
5 per side
	• Inhale and exhale between each movement
	
	• On each exhale, do a core drill (Kegel, then belly button pull)
	
	• On each inhale, relax core (abdominal muscles and Kegel)
	
	• During:
	
	  1. 1st Exhale and core drill: Lift your whole foot 1 inch off the mat
	  2. 2nd Exhale and core drill: Lower your foot
	
	• Continue steps 1–2 to alternate sides for 5 reps per side	

Core Drill Exercise— Supine Arm Pull
 	
5 per side
	• Inhale and exhale between each movement
	
	• On each exhale, do a core drill (Kegel, then belly button pull)
	
	• On each inhale, relax core (abdominal muscles and Kegel)
	
	• During:
	
	  1. 1st Exhale and core drill: Lift both arms straight out in front of you with elbows locked
	  2. 2nd Exhale and core drill: Use your shoulders to push one arm towards the ceiling and pull the other one back into the floor, then switch them
	
	• Repeat step 2 for 5 reps per side	

	Circuit: Do all 3 exercises in order, and repeat 2 more times for a total of 3 rounds		
Prone Lat Lift **15 per side**	• Start with your hand about 6 inches away from your body with your palm facing your hip • Lift your arm back and in, turning your palm up • Keep your elbow straight • At the top of each repetition, your hand should be directly over your hip		
Prone Rows **15 reps**	• Lie on your belly with your pillow under your lower chest and arms stretched out in front of you • Pull your arms back as you lift your head and chest up to row • Keep your feet on the mat the whole time		

Note: If it is still uncomfortable to lie on your belly, you may need to start on a softer surface, like a bed, at first.

Calf Raises **25 reps** **10 pulses**	• Hold on to a chair for balance • Come all the way up onto tiptoes slowly for 25 reps • Do 10 quick pulses from the halfway up position to the full up position		

STOP: Take a break to get some water between rounds. Repeat the circuit for 2 more rounds.

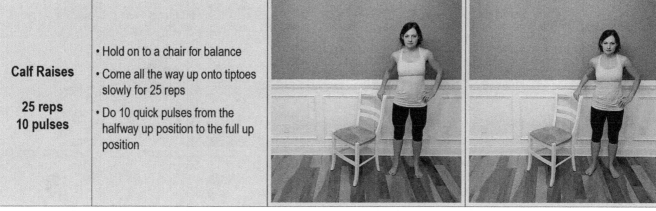

Light Stretching		
Calf Stretch **15 sec. per side**	• Stand stagger-step, and hold on for balance • Bend your front knee • Keep your back heel on the ground • Feel the stretch in your calf	
Thigh + Low Calf Stretch **15 sec. per side**	• Keep the stagger-step position • Bend your back knee • Release your heel from the floor • Tuck your butt under • Feel the stretch in the front of your hip and thigh and in your low calf	
Hamstring Stretch **15 sec. per side**	• Prop your heel forward • Pull your hips back • Keep the small of your back arched • Feel the stretch in the back of your thigh	
Chin Tuck **10 reps**	• Pull your head straight back • Add a little extra pressure with your hand • Feel the stretch at the base of your skull	
Cat Stretch **20–30 sec. per side**	• Reach for the right side of the mat • Curve your body into a "C" as you sit back • Feel the stretch on your left side and lower back • Switch sides and repeat	

Level 2

Circuit B

Before starting Level 2, you should have mastered all of the exercises from Level 1. If not, continue Level 1 until you can do all of the exercises in Level 1 correctly and without taking mid-set breaks.

Alternate Circuit A one day and Circuit B the next day for an 18–24 minute workout 4–6 times a week.

You Will Need:

- 24 Minutes
- A mat
- Water
- A towel

Core Drill Exercises		
Core Drill Exercise— Supine March **5 per side**	• Inhale and exhale between each movement • On each exhale, do a core drill (Kegel, then belly button pull) • On each inhale, relax core (abdominal muscles and Kegel) • During: 1. 1st Exhale and core drill: Lift your whole foot 1 inch off the mat 2. 2nd Exhale and core drill: Lower your foot • Continue steps 1–2 to alternate sides for 5 reps per side	
Core Drill Exercise— Supine Arm Pull **5 per side**	• Inhale and exhale between each movement • On each exhale, do a core drill (Kegel, then belly button pull) • On each inhale, relax core (abdominal muscles and Kegel) • During: 1. 1st Exhale and core drill: Lift both arms straight out in front of you with elbows locked 2. 2nd Exhale and core drill: Use your shoulders to push one arm towards the ceiling and pull the other one back into the floor, then switch them • Repeat step 2 for 5 reps per side	

Circuit: Do all 3 exercises in order, and repeat 2 more times for a total of 3 rounds		
Panini Press **25 per side**	• Start with your body in an "L" shape • Lift your top leg as a whole • Lower to repeat 25 times	
Clamshells **25 per side**	• Start with your body in the fetal position • Open your knees, keeping your feet together like a clamshell • Lower to repeat 25 times	
All Fours Glute Lifts + Hamstring Curl **15 lifts and 10 curls per side**	• Start out on all fours • With knee bent, bring your leg all the way up, then back down • Do 15 reps • Bring your leg back up once more with your knee bent, then slowly straighten out your knee to do 10 hamstring curls	
STOP: Take a break to get some water between rounds. Repeat the circuit for 2 more rounds.		

100

Light Stretching		
Calf Stretch **15 sec. per side**	• Stand stagger-step, and hold on for balance • Bend your front knee • Keep your back heel on the ground • Feel the stretch in your calf	
Thigh + Low Calf Stretch **15 sec. per side**	• Keep the stagger-step position • Bend your back knee • Release your heel from the floor • Tuck your butt under • Feel the stretch in the front of your hip and thigh and in your low calf	
Hamstring Stretch **15 sec. per side**	• Prop your heel forward • Pull your hips back • Keep the small of your back arched • Feel the stretch in the back of your thigh	
Chin Tuck **10 reps**	• Pull your head straight back • Add a little extra pressure with your hand • Feel the stretch at the base of your skull	
Cat Stretch **20–30 sec. per side**	• Reach for the right side of the mat • Curve your body into a "C" as you sit back • Feel the stretch on your left side and lower back • Switch sides and repeat	

Level 3

Circuit A

Before starting Level 3, you should have mastered all of the exercises from Level 2. If not, continue Level 2 until you can do all of the exercises in Level 2 correctly without stopping to take mid-set breaks.

Alternate Circuit A one day and Circuit B the next day for a 26–28 minute workout 4–6 times a week.

You Will Need:

- 28 Minutes
- A mat
- Water
- A towel

Core Drill Exercises		

Core Drill Exercise— Toe Tap
 	
10 per side
	• Inhale and exhale between each movement
	
	• On each exhale, do a core drill
	
	• On each inhale, relax core
	
	• During:
	
	  1. 1st Exhale and core drill: Lift one leg until shin is parallel with mat, toes pointed
	  2. 2nd Exhale and core drill: Lift your other leg until your shin is parallel with the mat, toes pointed
	  3. 3rd Exhale and core drill: Lower one leg until toes tap the mat, then bring leg back up
	
	• Repeat step 3 to alternate sides for 10 reps per side	

Core Drill Exercise—Arm Pull
 	
10 per side
	• Inhale and exhale between each movement
	
	• On each exhale, do a core drill
	
	• On each inhale, relax core
	
	• During:
	  1. 1st Exhale and core drill: Lift both arms straight out in front of you with elbows locked
	  2. 2nd Exhale and core drill: Use your shoulders to push one arm towards the ceiling and pull the other one back into the floor, then switch them
	
	• Repeat step 2 to for 10 reps
		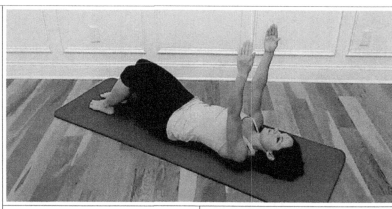
		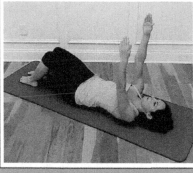 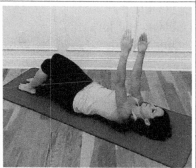

Circuit: Do all 5 exercises in order, and repeat 2 more times for a total of 3 rounds

Calf Raises **25 reps** **10 pulses**	• Hold on to a chair for balance • Come all the way up onto tiptoes slowly for 25 reps • Do 10 quick pulses from the halfway up position to the full up position	
Straight Leg Lifts **15 per side**	• Start with body and legs straight, hand on the mat for balance • Lift your top leg about 12 inches above your bottom leg • Don't roll your torso forward or back as you lift your leg • Lower to repeat 15 times	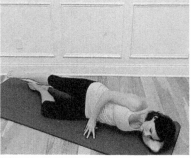 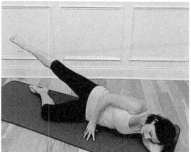
Diagonal Back Leg Lifts **15 per side**	• Bend your lower leg • Lift your top leg, this time bringing it slightly back, with your foot turned slightly out • Do 15 reps	

All Fours Glute Lift and Pulse + Hamstring Curl **15 lifts, 10 pulses, and 10 curls per side**	• Start out on all fours • Keeping your knee bent, lift your leg up and return to the start position for 15 reps • Pulse up towards the ceiling 10 times with your leg in the up position • Slowly straighten out your knee while holding your thigh up for 10 hamstring curls	
Hip Rotation in Side-lying **15 each way, each side**	• Start in the fetal position • Lift your top ankle, keeping your knees together • Do 15 reps • Bring your top leg out of the way by planting your foot behind your knee • Lift your bottom ankle, keeping your bottom thigh on the mat • Do 15 reps	

STOP: Take a break to get some water between rounds. Repeat the circuit for 2 more rounds.

Calf Stretch **15 sec. per side**	• Stand stagger-step, and hold on for balance • Bend your front knee • Keep your back heel on the ground • Feel the stretch in your calf	
Thigh + Low Calf Stretch **15 sec. per side**	• Keep the stagger-step position • Bend your back knee • Release your heel from the floor • Tuck your butt under • Feel the stretch in the front of your hip and thigh and in your low calf	
Hamstring Stretch **15 sec. per side**	• Prop your heel forward • Pull your hips back • Keep the small of your back arched • Feel the stretch in the back of your thigh	
Chin Tuck **10 reps**	• Pull your head straight back • Add a little extra pressure with your hand • Feel the stretch at the base of your skull	
Cat Stretch **20–30 sec. per side**	• Reach for the right side of the mat • Curve your body into a "C" as you sit back • Feel the stretch on your left side and lower back • Switch sides and repeat	

Level 3

Circuit B

Before starting Level 3, you should have mastered all of the exercises from Level 2. If not, continue Level 2 until you can do all of the exercises in Level 2 correctly without stopping to take mid-set breaks.

Alternate Circuit A one day and Circuit B the next day for a 26–28 minute workout 4–6 times a week.

You Will Need:

- 26 Minutes
- A mat
- Water
- A towel
- A pair of light (1–5 pound) hand weights
- A pillow (a nursing pillow works great)

Exercise Modifications
You should avoid the crunches and planks in this workout if either:
• You had a C-section and your doctor hasn't cleared you specifically to start crunches and planks.
OR
• You still have a separation (diastasis recti) of greater than two finger widths between your abdominal muscles (see p. 52 for diastasis recti self test). If you reach 8 weeks after having your baby and you still have a diastasis recti of greater than 2 finger widths, I recommend you see a physical therapist for an evaluation and hands-on, individualized instruction for progressing abdominal muscle work.
In the meantime, if either of the above apply to you, replace the crunches and planks in this workout with another round of the core drill exercises.

Core Drill Exercises		

Core Drill Exercise— Toe Tap
 	
10 per side
	• Inhale and exhale between each movement
	
	• On each exhale, do a core drill
	
	• On each inhale, relax core
	
	• During:
	
	  1. 1st Exhale and core drill: Lift one leg until shin is parallel with mat, toes pointed
	  2. 2nd Exhale and core drill: Lift your other leg until your shin is parallel with the mat, toes pointed
	  3. 3rd Exhale and core drill: Lower one leg until toes tap the mat, then bring leg back up
	
	• Repeat step 3 to alternate sides for 10 reps per side
		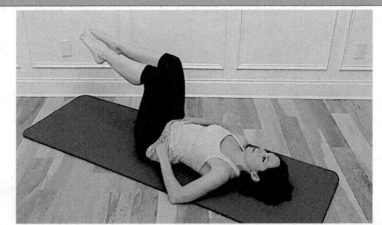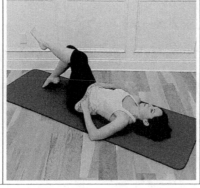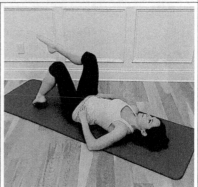

Core Drill Exercise—Arm Pull
 	
10 per side
	• Inhale and exhale between each movement
	
	• On each exhale, do a core drill
	
	• On each inhale, relax core
	
	• During:
	
	  1. 1st Exhale and core drill: Lift both arms straight out in front of you with elbows locked
	  2. 2nd Exhale and core drill: Use your shoulders to push one arm towards the ceiling and pull the other one back into the floor, then switch them
	
	• Repeat step 2 to for 10 reps
		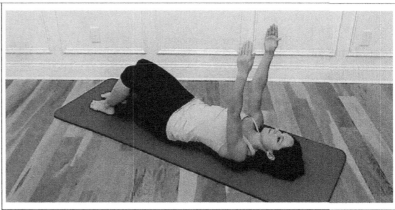
		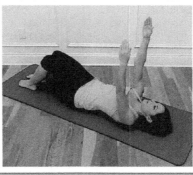 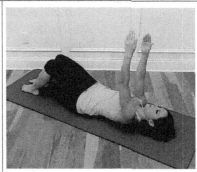

	**Circuit: Do all 6 exercises in order, and repeat 2 more times for a total of 3 rounds**	
Shoulder Blade Punch **30 reps**	• Hold your arms straight out in front of you, elbows locked • Quickly press the weights towards the ceiling by moving your shoulder blades out and around • Keep your elbows locked the whole time, using just your shoulders for the movement • Return to the start position to repeat 30 times	
Straight Leg Crunches **20 reps**	• Start with legs straight out in front of you, hands clasped behind your head • Crunch up so that the bottom tips of your shoulder blades are the only part of your shoulder blades touching the mat • Make sure not to pull on your neck to lift up • Keep your gaze 45 degrees in front of you	

Front Plank on Knees **20 sec.**	• Start on your knees and elbows • Lower your belly so that your shoulders, hips, and knees form a straight line • Hold 20 seconds	
Side Plank on Knees **20 sec. per side**	• Start with your body in an "L" shape • Lift up onto your elbow so that your shoulders, hips, and knees form a straight line • Hold 20 seconds, then switch sides	
Weighted Lat Lifts **15 per side**	• Holding a hand weight, start with your hand about 6 inches away from your body with your palm facing your hip • Lift your arm back and in, turning your palm up • Keep your elbow straight throughout the movement • At the top of each repetition, the hand weight should be directly over your hip	
Prone Rows **20 reps**	• Lie on your belly with your pillow under your lower chest and arms stretched out in front of you • Pull your arms back as you lift your head and chest up to row • Keep your feet on the mat the whole time	
Ws **15 reps**	• Lie on your belly with your pillow under your chest and your arms out to the side • Elbows should be bent at 90 degrees • Lift your hands up towards the ceiling (1–3 inches), moving just your forearms	

STOP: Take a break to get some water between rounds. Repeat the circuit for 2 more rounds.

Light Stretching		
Calf Stretch **15 sec. per side**	• Stand stagger-step, and hold on for balance • Bend your front knee • Keep your back heel on the ground • Feel the stretch in your calf	
Thigh + Low Calf Stretch **15 sec. per side**	• Keep the stagger-step position • Bend your back knee • Release your heel from the floor • Tuck your butt under • Feel the stretch in the front of your hip and thigh and in your low calf	
Hamstring Stretch **15 sec. per side**	• Prop your heel forward • Pull your hips back • Keep the small of your back arched • Feel the stretch in the back of your thigh	
Chin Tuck **10 reps**	• Pull your head straight back • Add a little extra pressure with your hand • Feel the stretch at the base of your skull	
Cat Stretch **20–30 sec. per side**	• Reach for the right side of the mat • Curve your body into a "C" as you sit back • Feel the stretch on your left side and lower back • Switch sides and repeat	

Level 4

Circuit A

Before starting Level 4, you should have mastered all of the exercises from Level 3. If not, continue Level 3 until you can do all of the exercises in Level 3 correctly without stopping to take mid-set breaks.

Alternate Circuit A one day and Circuit B the next day for a 27–32 minute workout 4–6 times a week.

You Will Need:

- 27 Minutes
- A mat
- Water
- A towel
- A chair
- A pair of light (1–5 pound) hand weights
- A pillow (a nursing pillow works great)

Exercise Modifications
You should avoid the crunches in this workout if either:
• You had a C-section and your doctor hasn't cleared you specifically to start crunches.
OR
• You still have a separation (diastasis recti) of greater than two finger widths between your abdominal muscles (see p. 52 for diastasis recti self test).
In the meantime, if either of the above apply to you, replace the crunches in this workout with another round of the core drill exercises.

Core Drill Exercises		

Core Drill Exercise— Slow Bicycling
 	
5 per side
	• Inhale and exhale between each movement
	• On each exhale, do a core drill
	• On each inhale, relax core
	• During:
	  1. 1st Exhale and core drill: Lift one leg and straighten it all the way out
	  2. 2nd Exhale and core drill: Bring your leg back to the start position
	• Alternate sides, repeating steps 1 and 2 for 5 per side	

Core Drill Exercise— Seated Row
 	
5 reps
	• Inhale and exhale between each movement
	
	• On each exhale, do a core drill
	
	• On each inhale, relax core
	
	• During:
	
	  1. 1st Exhale and core drill: Lift both arms straight out in front of you with elbows locked
	  2. 2nd Exhale and core drill: Pull your arms back into a high row
	  3. 3rd Exhale and core drill: Straighten arms
	
	• Repeat steps 2 and 3 for 5 reps		

Circuit: Do all 6 exercises in order, and repeat 2 more times for a total of 3 rounds			
Straight Leg Crunches **20 reps**	• Start with legs straight out in front of you, hands clasped behind your head • Crunch up so that the bottom tips of your shoulder blades are the only part of your shoulder blades touching the mat • Make sure not to pull on your neck to lift up • Keep your gaze 45 degrees in front of you		
Oblique Crunches **20 reps per side**	• Start with knees bent • Crunch up and twist • Do 20 to the right, then 20 to the left		
Weighted Lat Lifts **15 per side**	• Holding a hand weight, start with your hand about 6 inches away from your body with your palm facing your hip • Lift your arm back and in, turning your palm up • Keep your elbow straight throughout the movement • At the top of each repetition, the hand weight should be directly over your hip		
Ws **15 reps**	• Lie on your belly with your pillow under your chest and your arms out to the side • Elbows should be bent at 90 degrees • Lift your hands up towards the ceiling (1–3 inches), moving just your forearms		

Wall Push-Up with Plus **15 reps**	• Stand with feet 1–2 feet from the wall • Come down into a push-up on the wall • Return to the start position • Push your upper back out by moving your shoulder blades out and around • Return to start position	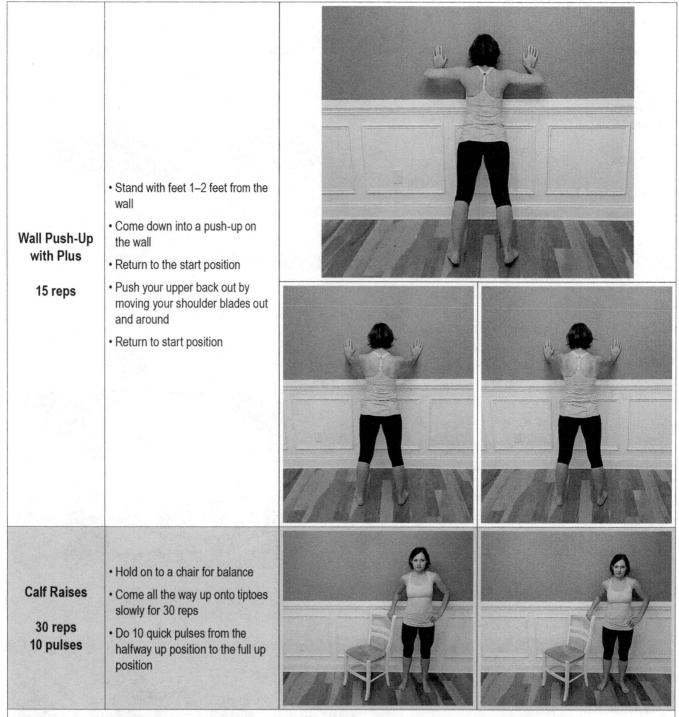
Calf Raises **30 reps** **10 pulses**	• Hold on to a chair for balance • Come all the way up onto tiptoes slowly for 30 reps • Do 10 quick pulses from the halfway up position to the full up position	

STOP: Take a break to get some water between rounds. Repeat the circuit for 2 more rounds.

Hamstring Stretch **20–30 sec. each side**	• Prop heel on chair or box • Keep back straight • Pull hips back to feel the stretch in the back of your thigh	
Corner Stretch **15–20 sec. twice**	• Lean into the doorway or corner until you feel a stretch in your chest • Switch your lead foot and repeat	
Chin Tuck **10 reps**	• Pull your head straight back • Add a little extra pressure with your hand • Feel the stretch at the base of your skull	
Figure 4 Stretch **20–30 sec. per side**	• Cross one ankle over the opposite knee and press your knee away from you using your hand • Switch sides and repeat	
Quad Stretch **20–30 sec. per side**	• Pull your ankle towards your butt (same arm, same leg)	

Level 4

Circuit B

Before starting Level 4, you should have mastered all of the exercises from Level 3. If not, continue Level 3 until you can do all of the exercises in Level 3 correctly without stopping to take mid-set breaks.

Alternate Circuit A one day and Circuit B the next day for a 27–32 minute workout 4–6 times a week.

You Will Need:

- 32 Minutes
- A mat
- Water
- A towel
- A chair

Exercise Modifications
You should avoid the planks in this workout if either: • You had a C-section and your doctor hasn't cleared you specifically to start planks. OR • You still have a separation (diastasis recti) of greater than two finger widths between your abdominal muscles (see p. 52 for diastasis recti self test). In the meantime, if either of the above apply to you, replace the planks in this workout with another round of the core drill exercises.

Core Drill Exercises		

Core Drill Exercise—Slow Bicycling
 	
5 per side
	• Inhale and exhale between each movement
	
	• On each exhale, do a core drill
	
	• On each inhale, relax core
	
	• During:
	
	  1. 1st Exhale and core drill: Lift one leg and straighten it all the way out
	
	  2. 2nd Exhale and core drill: Bring your leg back to the start position
	
	• Alternate sides, repeating steps 1 and 2 for 5 per side	

Core Drill Exercise— Seated Row
 	
 5 reps
	• Inhale and exhale between each movement
	
	 • On each exhale, do a core drill
	
	 • On each inhale, relax core
	
	 • During:
	
	   1. 1st Exhale and core drill: Lift both arms straight out in front of you with elbows locked
	   2. 2nd Exhale and core drill: Pull your arms back into a high row
	   3. 3rd Exhale and core drill: Straighten arms
	
	 • Repeat steps 2 and 3 for 5 reps	

Circuit: Do all 6 exercises in order, and repeat 2 more times for a total of 3 rounds

Front Plank on Knees **30 sec.**	• Start on your knees and elbows • Lower your belly so that your shoulders, hips, and knees form a straight line • Hold 30 seconds	
Side Plank on Knees **30 sec. per side**	• Start with your body in an "L" shape • Lift up onto your elbow so that your shoulders, hips, and knees form a straight line • Hold 30 seconds each side	
Hip Rotation in Side-lying **20 each way, each side**	• Start in the fetal position • Lift your top ankle, keeping your knees together • Do 20 reps • Bring your top leg out of the way by planting your foot behind your knee • Lift your bottom ankle, keeping your bottom thigh on the mat • Do 20 reps	

Long Glute Lift Plus Hamstring Curl **15 lifts** **10 curls**	• Start on all fours • Kick your leg straight behind you, straightening your knee, 15 times • Lift your leg again, this time with knee bent • Hold in the up position as you do 10 hamstring curls	
Diagonal Back Lifts **20 reps**	• Hold on to a chair for balance • Start with your leg out to the side, toes touching the floor • Lift out and slightly back with your toes turned slightly out • Tap toes back down between each rep	
Rear Leg Lifts **20 reps**	• Hold on to a chair for balance • Start with your leg behind you, toes touching the floor • Lift straight back, keeping leg totally straight and toes pointed • Tap toes back down between each rep	

STOP: Take a break to get some water between rounds. Repeat the circuit for 2 more rounds.

Hamstring Stretch **20–30 sec. each side**	• Prop heel on chair or box • Keep back straight • Pull hips back to feel the stretch in the back of your thigh	
Corner Stretch **15–20 sec. twice**	• Lean into the doorway or corner until you feel a stretch in your chest • Switch your lead foot and repeat	
Chin Tuck **10 reps**	• Pull your head straight back • Add a little extra pressure with your hand • Feel the stretch at the base of your skull	
Figure 4 Stretch **20–30 sec. per side**	• Cross one ankle over the opposite knee and press your knee away from you using your hand • Switch sides and repeat	
Quad Stretch **20–30 sec. per side**	• Pull your ankle towards your butt (same arm, same leg)	

Level 5

Circuit A

Before starting Level 5, you should have mastered all of the exercises from Level 4. If not, continue Level 4 until you can do all of the exercises in Level 4 correctly without stopping to take mid-set breaks.

Alternate Circuit A one day and Circuit B the next day for a 28–34 minute workout 4–6 times a week.

You Will Need:

- 34 Minutes
- A mat
- Water
- A towel
- A chair
- A pair of light (1–5 pound) hand weights

Exercise Modifications
You should avoid the crunches and planks in this workout if either:
• You had a C-section and your doctor hasn't cleared you specifically to start crunches and planks.
OR
• You still have a separation (diastasis recti) of greater than two finger widths between your abdominal muscles (see p. 52 for diastasis recti self test).
In the meantime, if either of the above apply to you, replace the crunches and planks in this workout with another round of the core drill exercises.

Core Drill Exercises		

Core Drill Exercise— Long Leg Bicycling
 	
5 per side
	• Inhale and exhale between each movement
	• On each exhale, do a core drill
	• On each inhale, relax core
	• During:
	  1. 1st Exhale and core drill: Bring one leg up with knee bent
	  2. 2nd Exhale and core drill: Bring second leg up with knee bent
	  3. 3rd Exhale and core drill: Straighten one leg to hover a few inches above the ground
	  4. 4th Exhale and core drill: Switch legs
	• Continue step 4 to alternate sides for 5 reps per side
		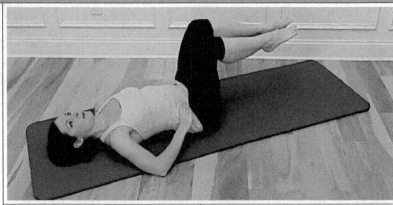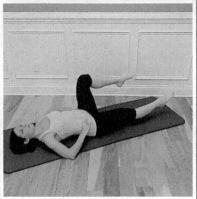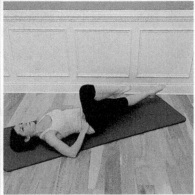

Core Drill Exercise— Seated Row
 	
10 reps
	• Inhale and exhale between each movement
	
	• On each exhale, do a core drill
	
	• On each inhale, relax core
	
	• During:
	
	  1. 1st Exhale and core drill: Lift arms straight out in front of you
	
	  2. 2nd Exhale and core drill: Pull arms back into a high row
	
	  3. 3rd Exhale and core drill: Straighten arms back out
	
	• Repeat steps 2 and 3 for 10 reps	

Circuit: Do all 7 exercises in order, and repeat 2 more times for a total of 3 rounds

Straight Leg Crunches **30 reps**	• Start with legs straight out in front of you, hands clasped behind your head • Crunch up so that the bottom tips of your shoulder blades are the only part of your shoulder blades touching the mat • Make sure not to pull on your neck to lift up • Keep your gaze 45 degrees in front of you	
Oblique Crunches **30 reps per side**	• Start with knees bent • Crunch up and twist • Do 30 to the right, then 30 to the left	
Half & Half Front Planks **10 sec. each side**	• Start in a front plank position on your knees with your shoulders, hips, and knees in a straight line • Straighten out one leg behind you, hovering your knee a few inches off the ground • Keep your pelvis level • Hold 10 seconds, then switch sides	

Side Plank on Knees **25 sec. per side**	• Start with your body in an "L" shape • Lift up onto your elbow so that your shoulders, hips, and knees form a straight line • Hold 25 seconds each side	
Ws **20 reps**	• Lie on your belly with your pillow under your chest and your arms out to the side • Elbows should be bent at 90 degrees • Lift your hands up towards the ceiling (1–3 inches), moving just your forearms	
Weighted Bird Dog, Arms Only **10 reps per side**	• Start on all fours, holding 1 pound hand weights • Slowly lift one arm at a time until it's straight with the rest of your body • Once your arm is straight, pull shoulder blade down away from your ear before switching sides	
Wall Push-Up with Plus **20 reps**	• Stand with feet 1–2 feet from the wall • Come down into a push-up on the wall • Return to the start position • Push your upper back out by moving your shoulder blades out and around • Return to start position	

STOP: Take a break to get some water between rounds. Repeat the circuit for 2 more rounds.

Hamstring Stretch **20–30 sec. each side**	• Prop heel on chair or box • Keep back straight • Pull hips back to feel the stretch in the back of your thigh	
Corner Stretch **15–20 sec. twice**	• Lean into the doorway or corner until you feel a stretch in your chest • Switch your lead foot and repeat	
Chin Tuck **10 reps**	• Pull your head straight back • Add a little extra pressure with your hand • Feel the stretch at the base of your skull	
Figure 4 Stretch **20–30 sec. per side**	• Cross one ankle over the opposite knee and press your knee away from you using your hand • Switch sides and repeat	
Quad Stretch **20–30 sec. per side**	• Pull your ankle towards your butt (same arm, same leg)	

Level 5

Circuit B

Before starting Level 5, you should have mastered all of the exercises from Level 4. If not, continue Level 4 until you can do all of the exercises in Level 4 correctly without stopping to take mid-set breaks.

Alternate Circuit A one day and Circuit B the next day for a 28–34 minute workout 4–6 times a week.

You Will Need:
- 28 Minutes
- A mat
- Water
- A towel
- A chair
- A pair of light (1–5 lb) hand weights

Core Drill Exercises		
Core Drill Exercise— Long Leg Bicycling **5 per side**	• Inhale and exhale between each movement • On each exhale, do a core drill • On each inhale, relax core • During: 1. 1st Exhale and core drill: Bring one leg up with knee bent 2. 2nd Exhale and core drill: Bring second leg up with knee bent 3. 3rd Exhale and core drill: Straighten one leg to hover a few inches above the ground 4. 4th Exhale and core drill: Switch legs • Continue step 4 to alternate sides for 5 reps per side	
Core Drill Exercise— Seated Row **10 reps**	• Inhale and exhale between each movement • On each exhale, do a core drill • On each inhale, relax core • During: 1. 1st Exhale and core drill: Lift arms straight out in front of you 2. 2nd Exhale and core drill: Pull arms back into a high row 3. 3rd Exhale and core drill: Straighten arms back out • Repeat steps 2 and 3 for 10 reps	

	Circuit: Do all 6 exercises in order, and repeat 2 more times for a total of 3 rounds	

Hip Lift Plus Rotation **20 reps per side**	• Start in fetal position • Lift your whole top leg up 6–12 inches • From there, do a quick kick with your ankle up towards the ceiling, moving just your lower leg • Bring your leg back down to the start position	
Rear Lunges **10 reps per side**	• Bring one leg back to lunge down • Alternate sides for 10 reps per side • Keep your back straight	
Rotational Front Leg Lifts **25 per side**	• Hold on to a chair for balance • Start with your leg out to the side, toes touching the floor • Bring your leg in and forward as you turn your foot out	
Side Leg Lifts **25 reps**	• Hold on to a chair for balance • Start with your leg out to the side, toes touching the floor • Lift out and slightly back with your toes turned slightly out • Tap toes back down between each rep	

Calf Raises **30 reps** **10 pulses**	• Hold on to a chair for balance • Come all the way up onto tiptoes slowly for 30 reps • Do 10 quick pulses from the halfway up position to the full up position		
Chair Squats **20 reps**	• Start standing 6–12 inches in front of a chair • Feet wider than shoulder width • Slide your hips back to allow your knees to bend • Squat back, bringing your arms straight out in front of you • Keep your weight through your heels and your knees behind your toes		

STOP: Take a break to get some water between rounds. Repeat the circuit for 2 more rounds.

124

Hamstring Stretch **20–30 sec. each side**	• Prop heel on chair or box • Keep back straight • Pull hips back to feel the stretch in the back of your thigh	
Corner Stretch **15–20 sec. twice**	• Lean into the doorway or corner until you feel a stretch in your chest • Switch your lead foot and repeat	
Chin Tuck **10 reps**	• Pull your head straight back • Add a little extra pressure with your hand • Feel the stretch at the base of your skull	
Figure 4 Stretch **20–30 sec. per side**	• Cross one ankle over the opposite knee and press your knee away from you using your hand • Switch sides and repeat	
Quad Stretch **20–30 sec. per side**	• Pull your ankle towards your butt (same arm, same leg)	

Level 6

Circuit A

Before starting Level 6, you should have mastered all of the exercises from Level 5. If not, continue Level 5 until you can do all of the exercises in Level 5 correctly without taking any breaks mid-set.

If you had a C-section, be sure your doctor has cleared you for all types of abdominal exercises before beginning this workout.

Alternate Circuit A one day and Circuit B the next day for a 30 minute workout 4–6 times a week.

You Will Need:

- 30 Minutes
- A mat
- Water
- A towel
- A pillow (a nursing pillow works great)

Modified Workout for Diastasis Recti
If you have a diastasis recti of more than two centimeters (or two finger widths), you'll need a hands-on evaluation from a physical therapist to determine exactly how to progress your abdominal muscle training in a way that's right for your body.
Since this workout is almost entirely comprised of exercises that challenge your abdominal muscles, do the following modified workout if you have a diastasis recti of more than 2 finger widths:
• Repeat 2 rounds of the core drill exercises (below)
• Repeat 3 alternating rounds of "Ws" and "Bird Dog" exercises (below)
• Cool down (below)

Dynamic Warm Up		

Core Drill Exercise— Diagonal Leg Lift
 	
5 per side
	• Inhale and exhale between each movement
	
	• On each exhale, do a core drill
	
	• On each inhale, relax core
	
	• During:
	
	  1. 1st Exhale and core drill: Draw one leg diagonally up, bringing your ankle in and bending your knee
	  2. 2nd Exhale and core drill: Bring your leg diagonally down and out, straightening your knee
	
	• Continue steps 1 and 2 for 5 reps, then repeat 5 reps on the other side	

Core Drill Exercise— Diagonal Arm Lift
 	
5 per side
	• Inhale and exhale between each movement
	
	• On each exhale, do a core drill
	
	• On each inhale, relax core
	
	• During:
	
	  1. 1st Exhale and core drill: Move your hand diagonally up above your head as you turn your palm towards you
	  2. 2nd Exhale and core drill: Move your arm diagonally back out to the side, turning your palm away from you
	
	• Repeat steps 1 and 2 for 5 reps, then repeat 5 reps on the other side		

	**Circuit: Do all 7 exercises in order, and repeat 2 more times for a total of 3 rounds**		
Ws **25 reps**	• Lie on your belly with your pillow under your chest and your arms out to the side • Elbows should be bent at 90 degrees • Lift your hands up towards the ceiling (1–3 inches), moving just your forearms		
Front Plank on Toes **15 sec.**	• Plank on toes and elbows • Body straight from shoulders to hips to knees to ankles • Hold 15 seconds		
Side Plank on Feet **15 sec. per side**	• Plank on side from elbow to feet • Body straight from shoulders to hips to knees to ankles • Hold 15 seconds per side		
Shoulder Blade Press on Knees **20 reps**	• Start in front plank position on knees • Press upper back up towards ceiling, higher than shoulder blades • Drop upper back lower than shoulder blades • Repeat 20 reps		

Bird Dog **10 per side**	• Start on all fours • Slowly lift one arm and the opposite leg to make a straight line from fingers to toes • In the up position, draw your shoulder blade down away from your ear • Switch sides and repeat	
Straight Leg Crunches **30 reps**	• Start with legs straight out in front of you, hands clasped behind your head • Crunch up so that the bottom tips of your shoulder blades are the only part of your shoulder blades touching the mat • Do not pull on your neck to lift up • Keep your gaze 45 degrees out in front of you	
Advanced Oblique Crunches with Leg Up **20 each side**	• Start with legs more than shoulder width apart • Lift your right leg up and out to the side with your knee bent • Crunch toward your right knee • Hold your right leg up for all 20 reps • Do 20 reps on the right, then 20 on the left • Keep your pelvis stable and on the mat throughout the whole exercise	

STOP: Take a break to get some water between rounds. Repeat the circuit for 2 more rounds.

Light Stretching		
Corner Stretch 15–20 sec. twice	• Lean into the doorway or corner until you feel a stretch in your chest • Switch your lead foot and repeat	
Hamstring Stretch 20–30 sec. each side	• Prop heel on chair or box • Keep back straight • Pull hips back to feel the stretch in the back of your thigh	
Neck Stretch 20–30 sec.	• Gently pull your nose towards your armpit • Feel the stretch at the base of your skull, the top of your shoulder blade, and in the middle of your back • Adjust the feel of this stretch by turning your head until it feels just right	
Figure 4 Stretch 20–30 sec. per side	• Cross one ankle over the opposite knee and press your knee away from you using your hand • Switch sides and repeat	
IT Band Stretch 20–30 sec. per side	• Cross your left ankle over your right knee • Let your body drop down to the left • Feel the stretch on the outside of your hip	
Quad Stretch 20–30 sec. per side	• Pull your ankle towards your butt (same arm, same leg)	

Level 6

Circuit B

Before starting Level 6, you should have mastered all of the exercises from Level 5. If not, continue Level 5 until you can do all of the exercises in Level 5 correctly without taking any breaks mid-set.

Alternate Circuit A one day and Circuit B the next day for a 30 minute workout 4–6 times a week.

You Will Need:

- 30 Minutes
- A mat
- Water
- A towel
- A chair

Core Drill Exercises		

Core Drill Exercise— Diagonal Leg Lift
 	
5 per side
	• Inhale and exhale between each movement
	• On each exhale, do a core drill
	• On each inhale, relax core
	• During:
	  1. 1st Exhale and core drill: Draw one leg diagonally up, bringing your ankle in and bending your knee
	  2. 2nd Exhale and core drill: Bring your leg diagonally down and out, straightening your knee
	• Continue steps 1 and 2 for 5 reps, then repeat 5 reps on the other side	

Core Drill Exercise— Diagonal Arm Lift
 	
5 per side
	• Inhale and exhale between each movement
	• On each exhale, do a core drill
	• On each inhale, relax core
	• During:
	  1. 1st Exhale and core drill: Move your hand diagonally up above your head as you turn your palm towards you
	  2. 2nd Exhale and core drill: Move your arm diagonally back out to the side, turning your palm away from you
	• Repeat steps 1 and 2 for 5 reps, then repeat 5 reps on the other side	

Circuit: Do all 6 exercises in order, and repeat 2 more times for a total of 3 rounds

Hip Lift Plus Rotation Pulse **20 lifts + 20 pulses per side**	• Start in fetal position • Lift your whole top leg up 6–12 inches • Return to the start position for 20 reps • Lift up again and do a quick kick with your ankle up towards the ceiling, moving just your lower leg • Hold your leg up to pulse up with just your lower leg for 20 reps	
Rotational Front Leg Lifts **30 per side**	• Hold on to a chair for balance • Start with your leg out to the side, toes touching the floor • Bring your leg in and forward as you turn your foot out	
Rear Lunges **15 reps per side**	• Bring your leg back to lunge down • Alternate sides for 15 reps per side • Keep your back straight	
Chair Squats **25 reps**	• Start standing 6–12 inches in front of a chair • Feet wider than shoulder width • Slide your hips back to allow your knees to bend • Squat back, bringing your arms straight out in front of you • Keep your weight through your heels and your knees behind your toes	

Single Leg Calf Raises **20 reps per side**	• Hold on to a chair for balance • On one leg, come up on to your tiptoes • Don't hike your hip as you get tired		
Side to Side Squat **10 per side**	• Move your right leg out to the side first to do a wide squat • Return to the center as you come back up • Step out to the left to do a wide squat • Return to the center as you come back up		

STOP: Take a break to get some water between rounds. Repeat the circuit for 2 more rounds.

	Light Stretching	
Corner Stretch 15–20 sec. twice	• Lean into the doorway or corner until you feel a stretch in your chest • Switch your lead foot and repeat	
Hamstring Stretch 20–30 sec. each side	• Prop heel on chair or box • Keep back straight • Pull hips back to feel the stretch in the back of your thigh	
Neck Stretch 20–30 sec.	• Gently pull your nose towards your armpit • Feel the stretch at the base of your skull, the top of your shoulder blade, and in the middle of your back • Adjust the feel of this stretch by turning your head until it feels just right	
Figure 4 Stretch 20–30 sec. per side	• Cross one ankle over the opposite knee and press your knee away from you using your hand • Switch sides and repeat	
IT Band Stretch 20–30 sec. per side	• Cross your left ankle over your right knee • Let your body drop down to the left • Feel the stretch on the outside of your hip	
Quad Stretch 20–30 sec. per side	• Pull your ankle towards your butt (same arm, same leg)	

Level 7

Circuit A

Before starting Level 7, you should have mastered all of the exercises from Level 6. If not, continue Level 6 until you can do all of the exercises in Level 6 correctly and without taking any mid-set breaks.

If you had a C-section, be sure your doctor has cleared you for all types of abdominal exercises before beginning this workout.

Alternate Circuit A one day and Circuit B the next day for a 23–33 minute workout 4–6 times a week.

You Will Need:

- 33 Minutes
- A mat
- Water
- A towel
- A pair of light (1–5 pound) hand weights

Modified Workout for Diastasis Recti		
If you have a diastasis recti of more than two centimeters (or two finger widths), you'll need a hands-on evaluation from a physical therapist to determine exactly how to progress your abdominal muscle training in a way that's right for your body. Since this workout is almost entirely comprised of exercises that challenge your abdominal muscles, do the following modified workout if you have a diastasis recti of more than 2 finger widths: • Repeat 2 rounds of the core drill exercises (below) • Repeat 3 alternating rounds of "Supine Hip External Rotation" and "Single Leg Run" exercises (below) • Cool down (below)		
Core Drill Exercises		
Core Drill Exercise— Wide Leg Squat **10 reps**	• Start with feet wider than shoulder width apart • Inhale and exhale between each movement • On each exhale, do a core drill • On each inhale, relax core • During: 　1. 1st Exhale and core drill: do a wide leg squat 　2. 1st Inhale: return to the start position • Repeat steps 1 and 2 for 10 reps	

Core Drill Exercise— Side Lean
 	
5 per side
	• Inhale and exhale between each movement
	• On each exhale, do a core drill
	• On each inhale, relax core
	• During:
	  1. 1st Exhale and core drill: Lift your arms out to the side
	  2. 2nd Exhale and core drill: Lean all the way to the right without losing balance, then return to center
	  3. 3rd Exhale and core drill: Lean all the way to the left without losing balance, then return to center
	• Repeat steps 2 and 3, alternating sides for 5 reps per side	

Circuit: Do all 7 exercises in order, and repeat 2 more times for a total of 3 rounds		
Shoulder Blade Press **25 reps**	• Start in front plank position on knees • Press upper back up towards ceiling, higher than shoulder blades • Drop upper back lower than shoulder blades • Repeat 25 reps	
Front Plank on Toes **15 sec.**	• Plank on toes and elbows • Body straight from shoulders to hips to knees to ankles • Hold 15 seconds	
Side Plank on Feet **15 sec. per side**	• Plank on side from elbow to feet • Body straight from shoulders to hips to knees to ankles • Hold 15 seconds per side	
Negative Sit- Ups **15 reps**	• Use your hands to pull yourself up into a sit-up • Cross arms over chest • Very slowly lower back to start position • Pull yourself back to the sit-up position	

Advanced Oblique Crunches with Toe Tap **20 each side**	• Start with legs more than shoulder width apart • Lift your right leg up and out to the side with your knee bent as you crunch up to the right knee • As you lower your torso back down, keep your knee bent and tap your toes on the mat • Do 20 reps on the right, then 20 on the left • Keep your pelvis stable and on the mat throughout the whole exercise	
Supine Hip External Rotation **20 reps per side**	• Start on your back in a figure 4 position • Hold your fist under your thigh for support • Lift your ankle up towards the ceiling, being careful not to lift your thigh off your fist as you lift	
Single Leg Running **10 per direction, per side**	• Stand on one leg, holding hand weights • Move arms as if running, allowing for natural body swing for 10 reps per side • Do 10 swings rotating your palms up each swing • Switch feet and repeat	

STOP: Take a break to get some water between rounds. Repeat the circuit for 2 more rounds.

Corner Stretch **15–20 sec. twice**	• Lean in to the doorway or corner until you feel a stretch in your chest • Switch your lead foot and repeat	
Hamstring Stretch **20–30 sec. each side**	• Prop heel on chair or box • Keep back straight • Pull hips back to feel the stretch in the back of your thigh	
Neck Stretch **20–30 sec.**	• Gently pull your nose towards your armpit • Feel the stretch at the base of your skull, the top of your shoulder blade, and in the middle of your back • Adjust the feel of this stretch by turning your head until it feels just right	
Figure 4 Stretch **20–30 sec. per side**	• Cross one ankle over the opposite knee and press your knee away from you using your hand • Switch sides and repeat	
IT Band Stretch **20–30 sec. per side**	• Cross your left ankle over your right knee • Let your body drop down to the left • Feel the stretch on the outside of your hip	
Quad Stretch **20–30 sec. per side**	• Pull your ankle towards your butt (same arm, same leg)	

Level 7

Circuit B

Before starting Level 7, you should have mastered all of the exercises from Level 6. If not, continue Level 6 until you can do all of the exercises in Level 6 correctly and without taking any mid-set breaks.

Alternate Circuit A one day and Circuit B the next day for a 23–33 minute workout 4–6 times a week.

You Will Need:

- 23 Minutes
- A mat
- Water
- A towel
- A chair
- A pair of light (1–5 pound) hand weights

Core Drill Exercises			

Core Drill Exercise— Wide Leg Squat
 	
 10 reps
	• Start with feet wider than shoulder width apart
	
	 • Inhale and exhale between each movement
	
	 • On each exhale, do a core drill
	
	 • On each inhale, relax core
	
	 • During:
	
	   1. 1st Exhale and core drill: do a wide leg squat and return to the start position
	  2. 1st Inhale: return to the start position
	
	 • Repeat steps 1 and 2 for 10 reps		

Core Drill Exercise— Side Lean
 	
 5 per side
	• Inhale and exhale between each movement
	
	 • On each exhale, do a core drill
	
	 • On each inhale, relax core
	
	 • During:
	
	   1. 1st Exhale and core drill: Lift your arms out to the side
	  2. 2nd Exhale and core drill: Lean all the way to the right without losing balance, then return to center
	  3. 3rd Exhale and core drill: Lean all the way to the left without losing balance, then return to center
	
	 • Repeat steps 2 and 3, alternating sides for 5 reps per side		

Circuit: Do all 6 exercises in order, and repeat 2 more times for a total of 3 rounds		
Bird Dog **10 per side**	• Start on all fours • Slowly lift one arm and the opposite leg to make a straight line from fingers to toes • In the up position, draw your shoulder blade down away from your ear • Switch sides and repeat	
Single Leg Calf Raises **25 reps per side**	• Hold on to a chair for balance • On one leg, come up on to your tiptoes • Don't hike your hip as you get tired	
Side to Side Squat **10 per side**	• Move your right leg out to the side first to do a wide squat • Return to the center as you come back up • Step out to the left to do a wide squat • Return to the center as you come back up	
Lateral Squat Jumps **10 per side**	• Move your right leg out to the side first to do a wide squat • Jump back to the center as you come back up • Step out to the left to do a wide squat • Jump back to the center as you come back up	

Forward Lunges **10 each side**	• Step forward to lunge down • Keep your back straight and your knee behind your toes • Alternate sides for 10 each side		
Lunge Ups **10 reps per side**	• Start in a split stance, holding hand weights • Drop down into a lunge • Push off your back leg to come up onto your lead leg only • Balance for a beat, then drop back down into your lunge to repeat • Do 10 on one side, then switch sides for 10 on the other side		

STOP: Take a break to get some water between rounds. Repeat the circuit for 2 more rounds.

Corner Stretch **15–20 sec. twice**	• Lean into the doorway or corner until you feel a stretch in your chest • Switch your lead foot and repeat	
Hamstring Stretch **20–30 sec. each side**	• Prop heel on chair or box • Keep back straight • Pull hips back to feel the stretch in the back of your thigh	
Neck Stretch **20–30 sec.**	• Gently pull your nose towards your armpit • Feel the stretch at the base of your skull, the top of your shoulder blade, and in the middle of your back • Adjust the feel of this stretch by turning your head until it feels just right	
Figure 4 Stretch **20–30 sec. per side**	• Cross one ankle over the opposite knee and press your knee away from you using your hand • Switch sides and repeat	
IT Band Stretch **20–30 sec. per side**	• Cross your left ankle over your right knee • Let your body drop down to the left • Feel the stretch on the outside of your hip	
Quad Stretch **20–30 sec. per side**	• Pull your ankle towards your butt (same arm, same leg)	

Level 8

Circuit A

Before starting Level 8, you should have mastered all of the exercises from Level 7. If not, continue Level 7 until you can do all of the exercises in Level 7 correctly without taking any breaks mid-set.

If you had a C-section, be sure your doctor has cleared you for all types of abdominal exercises before beginning this workout.

Alternate Circuit A one day and Circuit B the next day for a 27–29 minute workout 4–6 times a week.

You Will Need:
- 27 Minutes
- A mat
- Water
- A towel
- A pair of light (1–5 pound) hand weights

Modified Workout for Diastasis Recti
If you have a diastasis recti of more than two centimeters (or two finger widths), you'll need a hands-on evaluation from a physical therapist to determine exactly how to progress your abdominal muscle training in a way that's right for your body.
Since this workout is almost entirely comprised of exercises that challenge your abdominal muscles, do the following modified workout if you have a diastasis recti of more than 2 finger widths:
• Repeat 3 rounds of the core drill exercises (below), holding light 1–5 pound hand weights for the "Standing Diagonal Arm Lift" core drill exercise
• Cool down (below)

Core Drill Exercises		
Core Drill Exercise— Standing Diagonal Leg Lift **5 per side**	• Start with one leg out to the side, toes pointed and touching the ground • Inhale and exhale between each movement • On each exhale, do a core drill • On each inhale, relax core • During: 1. 1st Exhale and core drill: lift your leg diagonally up, bringing your hip out and your ankle in 2. 2nd Exhale and core drill: straighten your leg diagonally, back to the start position • Repeat steps 1 and 2 for 5 reps, then switch sides	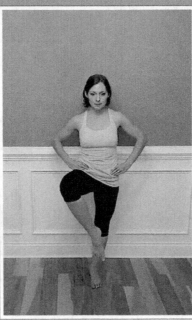 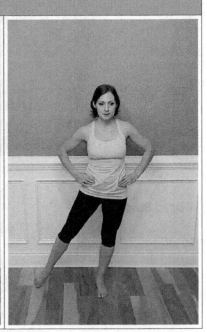

142

Core Drill Exercise—Standing Diagonal Arm Lift
 	
10 reps
	• Start with your palms back, arms 6–12 inches from your body
	• Inhale and exhale between each movement
	• On each exhale, do a core drill
	• On each inhale, relax core
	• During:
	  1. 1st Exhale and core drill: Rotate your palms around as you lift both arms up and in to cross wrists above your head
	  2. 2nd Exhale and core drill: Turn palms back as you bring your arms back down
	• Repeat steps 1 and 2 for 10 reps	

Circuit: Do all 6 exercises in order, and repeat 2 more times for a total of 3 rounds

Push-Up Plus on Knees **15 reps**	• Start in push-up position on knees with arms straight • Come down into a push-up • Push up to start position • Press upper back up towards ceiling, higher than shoulder blades • Return to start position	
Front Plank on Toes **15 sec.**	• Plank on toes and elbows • Body straight from shoulders to hips to knees to ankles • Hold 15 seconds	
Side Plank on Feet **15 sec per side**	• Plank on side from elbow to feet • Body straight from shoulders to hips to knees to ankles • Hold 15 seconds per side	
Double Leg Curl **15 reps**	• Start with hands under butt for support • Tuck knees up • Straighten legs to hover over mat (the lower your legs hover, the harder this exercise gets)	

Advanced Oblique Crunches with Toe Tap **25 each side**	• Start with legs more than shoulder width apart • Lift your right leg up and out to the side with your knee bent as you crunch up to the right knee • As you lower your torso back down, keep your knee bent and tap your toes on the mat • Do 25 reps on the right, then 25 on the left • Keep your pelvis stable and on the mat throughout the whole exercise	
Weighted Diagonal Arms **10 reps**	• Start holding weights at your side, palms back • Lift hands diagonally in, up, and over your head to cross wrists above your head, turning your palms towards your face • Bring your arms back down as you rotate your palms around to face back	

STOP: Take a break to get some water between rounds. Repeat the circuit for 2 more rounds.

Light Stretching		
Corner Stretch 15–20 sec. twice	• Lean into the doorway or corner until you feel a stretch in your chest • Switch your lead foot and repeat	
Hamstring Stretch 20–30 sec. each side	• Prop heel on chair or box • Keep back straight • Pull hips back to feel the stretch in the back of your thigh	
Neck Stretch 20–30 sec.	• Gently pull your nose towards your armpit • Feel the stretch at the base of your skull, the top of your shoulder blade, and in the middle of your back • Adjust the feel of this stretch by turning your head until it feels just right	
Figure 4 Stretch 20–30 sec. per side	• Cross one ankle over the opposite knee and press your knee away from you using your hand • Switch sides and repeat	
IT Band Stretch 20–30 sec. per side	• Cross your left ankle over your right knee • Let your body drop down to the left • Feel the stretch on the outside of your hip	
Quad Stretch 20–30 sec. per side	• Pull your ankle towards your butt (same arm, same leg)	

Level 8

Circuit B

Before starting Level 8, you should have mastered all of the exercises from Level 7. If not, continue Level 7 until you can do all of the exercises in Level 7 correctly without taking any breaks mid-set.

Alternate Circuit A one day and Circuit B the next day for a 27–29 minute workout 4–6 times a week.

You Will Need:

- 29 Minutes
- A mat
- Water
- A towel
- One heavier 5–15 pound weight (or an old laundry detergent jug filled with water)

Core Drill Exercises		
Core Drill Exercise—Standing Diagonal Leg Lift **5 per side**	• Start with one leg out to the side, toes pointed and touching the ground • Inhale and exhale between each movement • On each exhale, do a core drill • On each inhale, relax core • During: 　1. 1st Exhale and core drill: lift your leg diagonally up, bringing your hip out and your ankle in 　2. 2nd Exhale and core drill: straighten your leg diagonally, back to the start position • Repeat steps 1 and 2 for 5 reps, then switch sides	
Core Drill Exercise—Standing Diagonal Arm Lift **10 reps**	• Start with your palms back, arms 6–12 inches from your body • Inhale and exhale between each movement • On each exhale, do a core drill • On each inhale, relax core • During: 　1. 1st Exhale and core drill: Rotate your palms around as you lift both arms up and in to cross wrists above your head 　2. 2nd Exhale and core drill: Turn palms back as you bring your arms back down • Repeat steps 1 and 2 for 10 reps	

	Circuit: Do all 6 exercises in order, and repeat 2 more times for a total of 3 rounds		
Fire Hydrant **15 per side**	• Start on hands and knees • Keeping your knee bent, lift your leg out to the side as high as you can • Do 15 reps on one side, then switch sides for 15 more		
Side Plank with Leg Lift **5 reps per side**	• Start in side plank position • Lift your top leg 12 inches above your bottom leg • Don't let your hips drop down—keep your body straight • Hold 1 second, then return to the start position		
Squats with Weight **20 reps**	• Stand with feet wider than shoulder width, holding heavier weight • Slide your hips back to allow your knees to bend • Keep your back straight • Keep your knees behind your toes • Drive through your heels to come back up		
Calf Raises with Weight **20 reps**	• Stand holding heavier weight • Come up on your tiptoes as high as you can		
Forward Lunges **15 each side**	• Step far forward to lunge • Keep your knee behind your toes • Push off lead leg to return to start position • Alternate sides for 15 per side		
Scorpion Lunges **20 per side**	• Start with feet shoulder width apart • Step back as if you're doing a reverse lunge, but reach diagonally back to the opposite side • Drive through lead leg to return to start position • Alternate sides for 20 per side		
STOP: Take a break to get some water between rounds. Repeat the circuit for 2 more rounds.			

	Light Stretching	
Corner Stretch 15–20 sec. twice	• Lean in to the doorway or corner until you feel a stretch in your chest • Switch your lead foot and repeat	
Hamstring Stretch 20–30 sec. each side	• Prop heel on chair or box • Keep back straight • Pull hips back to feel the stretch in the back of your thigh	
Neck Stretch 20–30 sec.	• Gently pull your nose towards your armpit • Feel the stretch at the base of your skull, the top of your shoulder blade, and in the middle of your back • Adjust the feel of this stretch by turning your head until it feels just right	
Figure 4 Stretch 20–30 sec. per side	• Cross one ankle over the opposite knee and press your knee away from you using your hand • Switch sides and repeat	
IT Band Stretch 20–30 sec. per side	• Cross your left ankle over your right knee • Let your body drop down to the left • Feel the stretch on the outside of your hip	
Quad Stretch 20–30 sec. per side	• Pull your ankle towards your butt (same arm, same leg)	

Level 9

Circuit A

Before starting Level 9, you should have mastered all of the exercises from Level 8. If not, continue Level 8 until you can do all of the exercises in Level 8 correctly without taking any breaks mid-set.

If you had a C-section, be sure your doctor has cleared you for all types of abdominal exercises before beginning this workout.

Alternate Circuit A one day and Circuit B the next day for a 31–33 minute workout 4–6 times a week.

You Will Need:
- 33 Minutes
- A mat
- Water
- A towel
- A pair of light (1–5 pound) hand weights

Modified Workout for Diastasis Recti
If you have a diastasis recti of more than two centimeters (or two finger widths), you'll need a hands-on evaluation from a physical therapist to determine exactly how to progress your abdominal muscle training in a way that's right for your body. Since this workout is almost entirely comprised of exercises that challenge your abdominal muscles, do the following modified workout if you have a diastasis recti of more than 2 finger widths: • Repeat 3 rounds of the core drill exercises (below), holding light 1–5 pound hand weights for the "Slim Stance Diagonal Arms" core drill exercise • Cool down (below)

Core Drill Exercises		

Core Drill Exercise—Slim Lunge
 	
5 per side
	• Start stagger step, with one leg far in front of the other, in line as if on a balance beam
	
	• Inhale and exhale between each movement
	
	• On each exhale, do a core drill
	
	• On each inhale, relax core
	
	• During:
	  1. 1st Exhale and core drill: Lunge down
	  2. 1st Inhale: Return to standing
	
	• Repeat steps 1 and 2 for 5 reps, then switch sides
		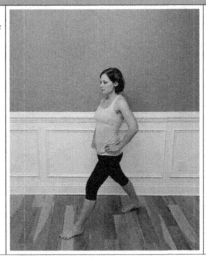	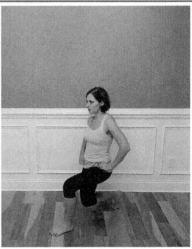

Core Drill Exercise— Slim Stance Diagonal Arms
 	
5 per side
	• Start stagger step, with one leg in front of the other, in line as if on a balance beam, with arms 6 inches from your body, palms back
	
	• Inhale and exhale between each movement
	
	• On each exhale, do a core drill
	
	• On each inhale, relax core
	
	• During:
	
	  1. 1st Exhale and core drill: Rotate your palms around as you lift both arms up and in to cross wrists above your head
	  2. 2nd Exhale and core drill: Turn palms back as you bring your arms back down
	
	• Repeat steps 1 and 2 for 5 reps, then switch your lead leg for 5 more reps	

Circuit: Do all 7 exercises in order, and repeat 2 more times for a total of 3 rounds

Push-Up Plus on Knees **20 reps**	• Start in push-up position on knees with arms straight • Come down into a push-up • Push up to start position • Press upper back up towards ceiling, higher than shoulder blades • Return to start position	
Front Plank on Toes **30 sec.**	• Start on toes and elbows • Make your body into a straight line from shoulders to hips to knees to ankles • Hold 30 seconds	
Side Plank on Feet **30 sec. per side**	• Plank on side from elbow to feet • Body straight from shoulders to hips to knees to ankles • Hold 30 seconds per side	

Double Leg Curl **20 reps**	• Start with hands under butt for support • Tuck knees up • Straighten legs to hover over mat (the lower your legs hover, the harder this exercise gets)		
Advanced Oblique Crunches with Leg Up **30 each side**	• Start with legs more than shoulder width apart • Lift your right leg up and out to the side with your knee bent • Crunch toward your right knee • Hold your right leg up for all 30 reps • Do 30 reps on the right, then 30 on the left • Keep your pelvis stable and on the mat throughout the whole exercise		
Side Plank with Leg Lift on Pillow **5 per side**	• Start in side plank with feet on pillow • Lift top leg 12 inches above bottom leg • Hold 1 second, then return to start position		
Weighted Diagonal Arms **10 each direction**	**1st Direction:** • Start holding weights at your side, palms back • Lift hands diagonally in, up, and over your head to cross wrists above your head, turning your palms towards your face • Do 10 this direction **2nd Direction:** • Start with wrists crossed at your waist, palms facing each other • Rotate your wrists around as you lift up and out • Do 10 this direction		

STOP: Take a break to get some water between rounds. Repeat the circuit for 2 more rounds.

Light Stretching		
Corner Stretch **15–20 sec. twice**	• Lean into the doorway or corner until you feel a stretch in your chest • Switch your lead foot and repeat	
Hamstring Stretch **20–30 sec. each side**	• Prop heel on chair or box • Keep back straight • Pull hips back to feel the stretch in the back of your thigh	
Neck Stretch **20–30 sec.**	• Gently pull your nose towards your armpit • Feel the stretch at the base of your skull, the top of your shoulder blade, and in the middle of your back • Adjust the feel of this stretch by turning your head until it feels just right	
Figure 4 Stretch **20–30 sec. per side**	• Cross one ankle over the opposite knee and press your knee away from you using your hand • Switch sides and repeat	
IT Band Stretch **20–30 sec. per side**	• Cross your left ankle over your right knee • Let your body drop down to the left • Feel the stretch on the outside of your hip	
Quad Stretch **20–30 sec. per side**	• Pull your ankle towards your butt (same arm, same leg)	

Level 9

Circuit B

Before starting Level 9, you should have mastered all of the exercises from Level 8. If not, continue Level 8 until you can do all of the exercises in Level 8 correctly without taking any breaks mid-set.

Alternate Circuit A one day and Circuit B the next day for a 31–33 minute workout 4–6 times a week.

You Will Need:
- 31 Minutes
- A mat
- Water
- A towel
- One heavier 5–15 pound weight or an empty laundry detergent jug filled with water

Core Drill Exercises			

Core Drill Exercise— Slim Lunge
 	
5 per side
	• Start stagger step, with one leg far in front of the other, in line as if on a balance beam
	
	• Inhale and exhale between each movement
	
	• On each exhale, do a core drill
	
	• On each inhale, relax core
	
	• During:
	  1. 1st Exhale and core drill: Lunge down
	  2. 2nd Inhale: Return to standing
	
	• Repeat steps 1 and 2 for 5 reps, then switch sides		

Core Drill Exercise— Slim Stance Diagonal Arms
 	
5 per side
	• Start stagger step, with one leg in front of the other, in line as if on a balance beam, with arms 6 inches from your body, palms back
	
	• Inhale and exhale between each movement
	
	• On each exhale, do a core drill
	
	• On each inhale, relax core
	
	• During:
	  1. 1st Exhale and core drill: Rotate your palms around as you lift both arms up and in to cross wrists above your head
	  2. 2nd Exhale and core drill: Turn palms back as you bring your arms back down
	
	• Repeat steps 1 and 2 for 5 reps, then switch your lead leg for 5 more reps		

Circuit: Do all 6 exercises in order, and repeat 2 more times for a total of 3 rounds

Fire Hydrant Kick **15 per side**	• Start on hands and knees • Keeping your knee bent, lift your leg out to the side as high as you can • Straighten your knee all the way • Bend your knee, then return to the start position • Do 15 reps on one side, then switch sides for 15 more	
Squats with Weight **30 reps**	• Stand with feet wider than shoulder width, holding heavier weight • Slide your hips back to allow your knees to bend • Keep your back straight • Keep your knees behind your toes • Drive through your heels to come back up	
Forward Lunges **20 each side**	• Step far forward to lunge • Keep your knee behind your toes • Push off lead leg to return to start position • Alternate sides for 20 per side	
Scorpion Lunges **25 per side**	• Start with feet shoulder width apart • Step back as if you're doing a reverse lunge, but reach diagonally back to the opposite side • Drive through lead leg to return to start position • Alternate sides for 25 per side	

Calf Raises with Weight **25 reps**	• Stand holding heavier weight • Come up on your tiptoes as high as you can		
Deadlifts **15 reps**	• Stand with feet wider than shoulder width • Hold your heavier weight in front of you with arms straight • Keep your back solid and straight • Hinge at the hips to bend forward, keeping your back straight • It's okay to let your knees bend a little as you go down		

STOP: Take a break to get some water between rounds. Repeat the circuit for 2 more rounds.

Corner Stretch 15–20 sec. twice	• Lean into the doorway or corner until you feel a stretch in your chest • Switch your lead foot and repeat	
Hamstring Stretch 20–30 sec. each side	• Prop heel on chair or box • Keep back straight • Pull hips back to feel the stretch in the back of your thigh	
Neck Stretch 20–30 sec.	• Gently pull your nose towards your armpit • Feel the stretch at the base of your skull, the top of your shoulder blade, and in the middle of your back • Adjust the feel of this stretch by turning your head until it feels just right	
Figure 4 Stretch 20–30 sec. per side	• Cross one ankle over the opposite knee and press your knee away from you using your hand • Switch sides and repeat	
IT Band Stretch 20–30 sec. per side	• Cross your left ankle over your right knee • Let your body drop down to the left • Feel the stretch on the outside of your hip	
Quad Stretch 20–30 sec. per side	• Pull your ankle towards your butt (same arm, same leg)	

Level 10

Circuit A

Before starting Level 10, you should have mastered all of the exercises from Level 9. If not, continue Level 9 until you can do all of the exercises in Level 9 correctly without taking any breaks mid-set.

Alternate Circuit A one day and Circuit B the next day for a 33–35 minute workout 4–6 times a week.

You Will Need:
- 35 Minutes
- A mat
- Water
- A towel
- A pillow
- 2 chairs
- Light (1–5 pound) hand weights
- One heavier 5–15 pound weight or an empty laundry detergent jug filled with water

Core Drill Exercises		
Core Drill Exercise— T-Stance **5 per side**	• Inhale and exhale between each movement • On each exhale, do a core drill • On each inhale, relax core • During: 1. 1st Exhale and core drill: Bring arms out to the side 2. 2nd Exhale and core drill: Stand on one leg, knee up 3. 3rd Exhale and core drill: Lower your torso until it's parallel with the ground and straighten out your back leg, then return to single leg position on inhale • Repeat step 3 for 5 reps, then switch sides	

Core Drill Exercise— Single Leg Diagonal Arms
 	
5 per side
	• Inhale and exhale between each movement
	• On each exhale, do a core drill
	• On each inhale, relax core
	• During:
	  1. 1st Exhale and core drill: Stand on one leg with hands about 6 inches from your side, palms back
	  2. 2nd Exhale and core drill: Rotate your palms around as you lift both arms up and in to cross wrists above your head
	  3. 3rd Exhale and core drill: Turn palms back as you bring your arms back down
	• Repeat steps 1 and 2 for 5 reps, then switch your lead leg for 5 more reps		

Circuit: Do all 7 exercises in order, and repeat 2 more times for a total of 3 rounds

Fire Hydrant Kick Lift **15 per side**	• Start on hands and knees • Keeping your knee bent, lift your leg out to the side as high as you can • Straighten your knee all the way • Lower your leg to tap your toes on the ground, then bring it back up • Bend your knee, then return to the start position • Do 15 reps on one side, then switch sides for 15 more		
Side Plank with Leg Lift on Pillow **5 per side**	• Start in side plank with your feet on a pillow • Lift top leg 12 inches above bottom leg • Hold 2 seconds, then return to start position		

Lateral Squat to Toes **10 each side**	• Start with feet wide apart, holding on to the chair next to you for balance • Squat down, and as you come up, lift onto one foot, up onto tiptoes • Drop back down into wide squat to repeat for 10 reps • Move the chair to the opposite side to repeat 10 on the other side		
Romanian Lunges **10 per side**	• Start with one foot far back on a chair behind you and holding a chair in front of you for balance • Hold a weight in your hand • As you lunge down, do a bicep curl with the weight • Keep your knee behind your toes of the lunging leg • Do 10 reps on one side, then switch sides		
Lateral Squat Jumps **15 per side**	• Move your right leg out to the side first to do a wide squat • Jump back to the center • Step out to the left to do a wide squat • Jump back to the center		
Lunge Ups **15 reps per side**	• Start in a split stance, holding hand weights • Drop down into a lunge • Push off your back leg to come up onto your lead leg only • Balance for a beat, then drop back down into your lunge to repeat • Do 10 on one side, then switch sides for 10 on the other side		
Deadlifts **20 reps**	• Stand with feet wider than shoulder width • Hold your heavier weight in front of you with arms straight • Keep your back solid and straight • Hinge at the hips to bend forward, keeping your back straight • It's okay to let your knees bend a little as you go down		

STOP: Take a break to get some water between rounds. Repeat the circuit for 2 more rounds.

Light Stretching		
Corner Stretch **15–20 sec. twice**	• Lean into the doorway or corner until you feel a stretch in your chest • Switch your lead foot and repeat	
Hamstring Stretch **20–30 sec. each side**	• Prop heel on chair or box • Keep back straight • Pull hips back to feel the stretch in the back of your thigh	
Neck Stretch **20–30 sec.**	• Gently pull your nose towards your armpit • Feel the stretch at the base of your skull, the top of your shoulder blade, and in the middle of your back • Adjust the feel of this stretch by turning your head until it feels just right	
Figure 4 Stretch **20–30 sec. per side**	• Cross one ankle over the opposite knee and press your knee away from you using your hand • Switch sides and repeat	
IT Band Stretch **20–30 sec. per side**	• Cross your left ankle over your right knee • Let your body drop down to the left • Feel the stretch on the outside of your hip	
Quad Stretch **20–30 sec. per side**	• Pull your ankle towards your butt (same arm, same leg)	

Level 10

Circuit B

Before starting Level 10, you should have mastered all of the exercises from Level 9. If not, continue Level 9 until you can do all of the exercises in Level 9 correctly without taking any breaks mid-set.

If you had a C-section, be sure your doctor has cleared you for all types of abdominal exercises before beginning this workout.

Alternate Circuit A one day and Circuit B the next day for a 33–35 minute workout 4–6 times a week.

You Will Need:

- 33 Minutes
- A mat
- Water
- A towel
- Light (1–5 pound) hand weights

Modified Workout for Diastasis Recti		
If you have a diastasis recti of more than two centimeters (or two finger widths), you'll need a hands-on evaluation from a physical therapist to determine exactly how to progress your abdominal muscle training in a way that's right for your body. Since this workout is almost entirely comprised of exercises that challenge your abdominal muscles, do the following modified workout if you have a diastasis recti of more than 2 finger widths: • Repeat 3 rounds of the core drill exercises (below), holding light 1–5 pound hand weights for the "Single Leg Diagonal Arms" core drill exercise • Cool down (below)		
Core Drill Exercises		

Core Drill Exercise— T-Stance
 	
5 per side
	• Inhale and exhale between each movement
	• On each exhale, do a core drill
	• On each inhale, relax core
	• During:
	  1. 1st Exhale and core drill: Bring arms out to the side
	  2. 2nd Exhale and core drill: Stand on one leg, knee up
	  3. 3rd Exhale and core drill: Lower your torso until it's parallel with the ground and straighten out your back leg, then return to single leg position on inhale
	• Repeat step 3 for 5 reps, then switch sides	

Core Drill Exercise— Single Leg Diagonal Arms
 	
5 per side
	• Inhale and exhale between each movement
	• On each exhale, do a core drill
	• On each inhale, relax core
	• During:
	  1. 1st Exhale and core drill: Stand on one leg with hands about 6 inches from your side, palms back
	  2. 2nd Exhale and core drill: Rotate your palms around as you lift both arms up and in to cross wrists above your head
	  3. 3rd Exhale and core drill: Turn palms back as you bring your arms back down
	
	• Repeat steps 1 and 2 for 5 reps, then switch your lead leg for 5 more reps		

Circuit: Do all 6 exercises in order, and repeat 2 more times for a total of 3 rounds

Side to side shoulder blade press **10 per side and middle**	• Start in front plank position on toes • Press your upper back towards the ceiling, then let it drop below your shoulder blades • Do 10 reps • Shift your weight over your right elbow and repeat for 10 reps • Shift your weight over your left elbow and repeat for 10 reps		
Rotational Side Plank **10 per side**	• Start in side plank • Bend your top knee slightly and pivot on your elbow to tap your knee on the mat, then return to your side plank • Do 10 reps, then switch sides for 10 more		

Front Plank with 3 Variations **1 round**	• Start in front plank position with shoulders, hips, knees, and ankles in a straight line • Hold 7 seconds • Glide your body forward on your toes • Hold 7 seconds • Glide your body back, past your original plank position • Hold 7 seconds • Place the tops of your feet on your mat • Hold 7 seconds		
Double Leg Lowering **15 reps**	• Start with hands under butt for support • Lift legs straight up • Lower legs to hover over mat (the lower your legs hover, the harder this exercise gets) • Lift legs straight back up		
Advanced Oblique Crunches with Leg Extension **30 each side**	• Start with legs more than shoulder width apart • Lift your right leg up and out to the side with your knee bent as you crunch up to the right knee • As you lower your torso back down, straighten your leg out and hover it above the mat • Do 30 reps on the right, then 30 on the left • Keep your pelvis stable and on the mat throughout the whole exercise		

163

Weighted Diagonal Arms **15 each direction**	**1st Direction:** • Start holding weights at your side, palms back • Lift hands diagonally in up and over your head to cross wrists above your head, turning your palms towards your face • Do 15 this direction **2nd Direction:** • Start with wrists crossed at your waist, palms facing each other • Rotate your wrists around as you lift up and out • Do 15 this direction	

STOP: Take a break to get some water between rounds. Repeat the circuit for 2 more rounds.

Corner Stretch **15–20 sec. twice**	• Lean into the doorway or corner until you feel a stretch in your chest • Switch your lead foot and repeat	
Hamstring Stretch **20–30 sec. each side**	• Prop heel on chair or box • Keep back straight • Pull hips back to feel the stretch in the back of your thigh	
Neck Stretch **20–30 sec.**	• Gently pull your nose towards your armpit • Feel the stretch at the base of your skull, the top of your shoulder blade, and in the middle of your back • Adjust the feel of this stretch by turning your head until it feels just right	
Figure 4 Stretch **20–30 sec. per side**	• Cross one ankle over the opposite knee and press your knee away from you using your hand • Switch sides and repeat	
IT Band Stretch **20–30 sec. per side**	• Cross your left ankle over your right knee • Let your body drop down to the left • Feel the stretch on the outside of your hip	
Quad Stretch **20–30 sec. per side**	• Pull your ankle towards your butt (same arm, same leg)	

Appendix A.

Walking Progression

Walking

Right after you have your baby, you may be waddling more than walking. Once you're home and recovering, start taking short walks with your stroller once or twice a day. Just go as far as is comfortable, which will likely be under a quarter mile for the first two weeks or so as your body is healing.

Once it's comfortable to walk, you can gradually pick up speed and add distance. When you can walk for 20 minutes at a solid pace fast enough that you could refer to it as "brisk," you're ready to start cardio training in earnest.

Increase your mileage (or time if you don't know the distance) by about 10 percent per week. It's best to make laps at first rather than go out and back in case you or your baby need to stop. A good goal for a brisk pace is 15 minutes per mile.

Stage	Walk	Pace
1	5-10 minutes	Slow, postpartum waddle
2	12 minutes	Comfortable slow pace
3	15 minutes	Comfortable pace
4	20 minutes	Comfortable pace
5	20 minutes	Brisk pace
6	22 minutes	Brisk pace
7	25 minutes	Brisk pace
8	28 minutes	Brisk pace
9	31 minutes	Brisk pace
10	35 minutes	Brisk pace

Appendix B.

Cycling Progression and Workouts

Cycling

If you have access to a spin bike, you can do workouts on your own as soon as your doctor clears you for cardiovascular exercise and you're walking 20 minutes at a brisk pace without difficulty. If you still have pain in your perineum, you can do a standing workout on the bike.

When biking on a spin bike, there shouldn't be bouncing—there should be enough resistance that you maintain a smooth ride. If you're bouncing, turn up the resistance.

Sidebar: I am fortunate enough to have my own spin bike, and it's my most important piece of gym equipment. If you find that the best way to get a solid cardio workout in is at home while your baby sleeps and you're looking at options, I recommend a spin bike. I also have a treadmill, but even as a competitive runner, I prefer my spin bike because it's simple, doesn't require electricity, has minimal maintenance requirements that even I can handle myself, provides a great workout, and doesn't make any noise (unfortunately me running on the treadmill wakes my son).

Cycling progression* (for trainer or spin bike):

*Position should be standing if your nether-region isn't quite ready for comfortable bike sitting. Progress to the next level only once you're able to maintain the target cadence range and it has become easy for you.

Stage	Bike	Cadence
1	5–10 minutes	60–80 RPMs
2	12 minutes	60–80 RPMs
3	15 minutes	70–80 RPMs
4	20 minutes	70–80 RPMs

Here are a few of my favorite on-your-own bike workouts once you've completed the above progression:

Standing workout (if your nether-region isn't quite ready for comfortable bike sitting):

Warm Up	Fast cadence (90–100 RPMs)	Moderate cadence (70–80 RPMs)	Repeat	Cool Down	Total Time
Standing	Standing	Standing	—	Standing	—
5 minutes	30 seconds	30 seconds	10 times	5 minutes	30 minutes

Two minute drills:

Warm Up	Fast cadence (90–100 RPMs)	Moderate cadence (70–80 RPMs)	Repeat	Cool Down	Total Time
Sitting	Sitting	Stand, then sit	—	Sitting	—
5 minutes	2 minutes	2 minutes	5–10 times	5 minutes	30–50 minutes

3-2-1 drills:

Work	Time	Position
Warm up	5 minutes	Sitting
Hill (increase resistance every 30 seconds until it's so heavy you have to stand to keep the wheels turning for the last minute)	3 minutes	Sit, then stand
Moderate cadence (70-80 RPMs)	3 minutes	Sitting
Fast cadence (90-100 RPMs)	2 minutes	Sitting
Moderate cadence (70-80 RPMs)	2 minutes	Sitting
Up-Downs (stand up for 4 steps, sit down for 4 steps, with heavy resistance)	1 minute	Sit/stand
Moderate cadence (70-80 RPMs)	1 minute	Sitting
Repeat 3-2-1s for 2 total rounds		
Cool Down	5 minutes	Sitting
Total Time	**40 minutes**	

Appendix C.

Ready to Run?

Running

Checklist
- ☐ My doctor has cleared me to start running
- ☐ I am exercising and walking without any pain
- ☐ I have a good pair of running shoes (and I'm not just dusting off the same exact pair of running shoes I had before I got pregnant)
- ☐ I am at least a Level 3 on the Sahrmann's core strength test below

Before you start a run progression, you need to be able to stabilize your core as you move your legs. The Sahrmann core test is a great way to check to see if you're ready. You'll need to be at least a Level 3 on her scale. I recommend wearing socks during this test so that your feet will slide. This is a progressive test, so you don't stop between levels— you just keep going until you reach Level 3 or you stop if you can't keep your back and pelvis perfectly steady.

Sahrmann Core Test
Start position: Start out lying on your back with your knees bent and feet flat. You can place a rolled towel under your head for support for your neck.

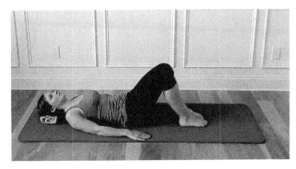

Getting ready: Place your hands at the small of your back so that you can feel the pressure of your back on your hands. Rock your pelvis forward and back to find a comfortable neutral position, then do your core drill for a practice run.

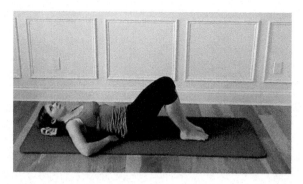

Take a deep wide rib breath in, then on exhale contract pelvic floor, and move right into your belly button pull. Once you feel your core contraction, take note of the pressure on your hands. During the test you'll have to keep the pressure the same on both hands throughout the movements. If you feel a difference side to side, or you're unable to keep from rocking as you move your legs, stop there. You have to get to Level 3 to start the run progression. When you get your core contraction for the test, instead of relaxing your muscles to reset for each breath, we're going to hold your core contraction but *keep breathing normally* through the test.

Level 1: When you're ready, start your core drill again. Once you feel your core kick in, lift your right foot off the ground so that your knee comes up just past your hip. Bring the other leg up with it. Did the pressure under your hands remain the same side to side? If so, you passed Level 1, so keep holding. If not, put your feet down, and keep working with the program for another week, then test again.

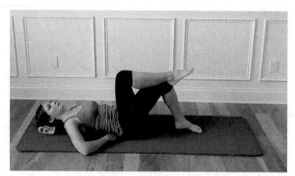
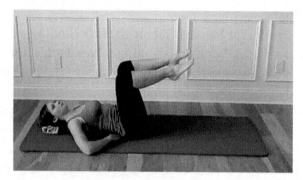

Level 2: Now bring your right heel down to the mat and glide it along the mat until your leg is straight. Pull it back the same way in reverse to the up position. Repeat on the left. Did the pressure under your hands remain the same side to side? If so, you passed Level 2, so keep holding. If not, put your feet down, and keep working with the program for another week, then test again.

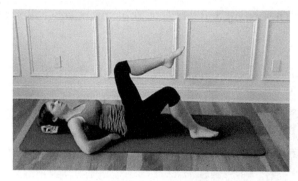
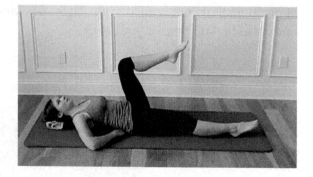

Level 3: Now bring your right heel to about 6 inches above the mat, straighten it out, and bring it all the way back in. Repeat on the left. Did the pressure under your hands remain the same side to side? If so, you passed Level 3, and your core is ready to start a run progression.

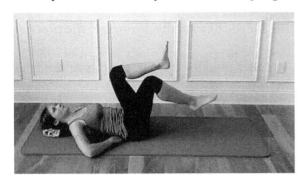 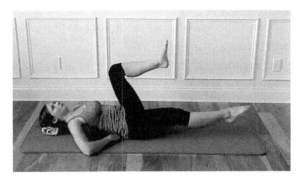

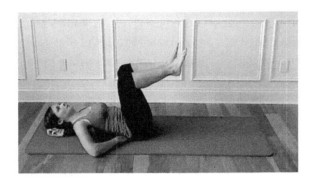

Run Progression Guidelines

On the tables below, do each level at least twice before progressing to the next level. You should do each level until it's comfortable and feels easy before progressing. This may take a week or two for some levels.

- If you experience any discomfort or pain, stop running for the day and back down to the previous level the next time you run.
- For example, if you get to Level 4 and experience symptoms, stop for the day, then two days later try Level 3 again.
- If you still experience pain, stop for a week. If it's still painful the next time you try, seek help from your physician or physical therapist.

Run no more than 3–4 times weekly.

Run Progressions

Please note: these levels do not correspond with the levels in your exercise program. It's very likely you won't be truly ready to start running until you are in Level 4 to Level 6 of your exercise program, and you don't have to progress levels of your run progression at the same rate you're progressing your exercise program. They're independent of each other.

Solo Run Progression (No Stroller)

Phase 1				
Level	**Walk**	**Run**	**Repetitions**	**Total Time**
1	4 minutes	1 minute	Repeat 5 times	25 minutes
2	3 minutes	2 minutes	Repeat 5 times	25 minutes
3	2 minutes	3 minutes	Repeat 5 times	25 minutes
4	1 minute	4 minutes	Repeat 5 times	25 minutes
Phase 2				
Level	**Walk**	**Run**	**Repetitions**	**Total Time**
5	5 minutes	10 minutes	5 minutes	20 minutes
6	3 minutes	14 minutes	3 minutes	20 minutes
7	1 minute	18 minutes	1 minute	20 minutes
8	3 minutes	20 minutes	2 minutes	25 minutes
9	1 minute	23 minutes	1 minute	25 minutes
10	—	25 minutes	—	25 minutes

After you reach Level 10, add 5 minutes every week or two to your run time until you reach your goal running duration.

Jogging Stroller Run Progression

When is it safe to take your baby out in a jogging stroller? Good question, and you'll find lots of authoritative-sounding answers on the internet. The generally accepted standard is that your baby is ready to ride as a passenger for a stroller run after they are six months old with good head control, but this recommendation was initially published in a running magazine years ago and has not been backed up by research.[39] That doesn't mean it's a bunch of bunk—it just means that it's not something that's been researched, probably because no parent is going to sign their baby up for a research study to see if something would or wouldn't harm them.

During the first six months of life, your baby should be rear-facing in an infant car seat with an appropriate car seat adapter whenever you walk with your baby in the jogging stroller. You'll have to be sure the car seat sits at an appropriately reclined position, just the same as in the car. This is to prevent your baby's head from nodding forward during a nap while you're walking (your baby may not have the strength to lift his or her head back up to breathe adequately if the seat is too upright). Check with your local fire station or police department (the same folks who do the car seat inspection in your car) to be sure you've got it right. During those first six months, when your baby is riding in the car seat attached to your jogging stroller, it's not safe to run with your baby in the jogging stroller because adding the car seat changes the center of gravity for the stroller. A higher center of gravity means that your stroller could tip over much more easily, especially when you go around curves, run on crowned roads, hit an errant rock or stick, or zip around corners.

Bottom line: ask your pediatrician before running with your baby in the jogging stroller. Write the question down and ask at one of your checkups. The answer depends on lots of individual factors such as your baby's status and health, your environment (traffic, weather, terrain), and your stroller. Be sure to write down and discuss each of those factors with your pediatrician. When your pediatrician does give you the green light, make sure to stick to smooth surfaces for younger babies, check that your stroller or insert offers adequate head support on the sides, and discuss the proper recline of the stroller seat with your pediatrician.

If you are running sometimes by yourself and at other times with your stroller, use the stroller running progression as a separate progression from the no-stroller progression. For example, if you're at Level 4 in the no-stroller progression when you get the green light from your pediatrician to start using a jogging stroller, start at Level 1 for the stroller progression anyway, and stay on track with your Level 4 program for the no-stroller progression. Running with a stroller, as you'll find out, is quite different in some ways from running solo, particularly for your upper body, and it takes a little getting used to.

Level	Walk	Run	Repetitions	Total Time
1	4 minutes	1 minute	Repeat 5 times	25 minutes
2	3 minutes	2 minutes	Repeat 5 times	25 minutes
3	2 minutes	3 minutes	Repeat 5 times	25 minutes
4	1 minute	4 minutes	Repeat 5 times	25 minutes
5	1 minute	5 minutes	Repeat 5 times	30 minutes
6	1 minute	10 minutes	Repeat 2 times	22 minutes
7	1 minute	15 minutes	Repeat 2 times	32 minutes
8	5 minutes	20 minutes	Do not repeat	25 minutes
9	5 minutes	25 minutes	Do not repeat	30 minutes
10	—	30 minutes	Do not repeat	30 minutes

After you reach Level 10, add 5 minutes every week or two to your run time until you reach your goal running duration.

References

1. ACOG Committee Opinion No. 650. *Obstetrics & Gynecology*. 2015;126(6):e135-e142.

2. Segal, N. A., E. R. Boyer, P. Teran-Yengle, N. A. Glass, H. J. Hillstrom, and H. J. Yack. "Pregnancy Leads to Lasting Changes in Foot Structure." American Journal of Physical Medicine & Rehabilitation 92, no. 3 (2013): 232-240.

3. Takeda, K. "A Kinesiological Analysis of the Stand-to-Sit during the Third Trimester." Journal of Physical Therapy Science 24 (2012): 621-624.

4. Gilleard, W. L. "Trunk motion and gait characteristics of pregnant women when walking: report of a longitudinal study with a control group." BMC Pregnancy and Childbirth 13, no. 71 (2013): 1-8.

5. Opala-Berdzik, A., B. Bacik, and M. Kurkowska. "Biomechanical changes in pregnant women." Physiotherapy 17, no. 3 (2009): 51-55.

6. Aldabe, D., S. Milosavljevic, and M. D. Bussey. "Is pregnancy related pelvic girdle pain associated with altered kinematic, kinetic and motor control of the pelvis? A systematic review." European Spine Journal 21, no. 9 (2012): 1777-1787.

7. Moore, K. L., A. F. Dalley, and A. M. R. Agur. Clinically Oriented Anatomy. Baltimore: Lippincott Williams & Wilkins, 1999.

8. Smith, M. D., M. W. Coppieters, P. W. Hodges. "Postural activity of the pelvic floor muscles is delayed during rapid arm movements in women with stress urinary incontinence." International Urogynecology Journal 18 (2007): 901-911.

9. Hodges, P. W., and R. Sapsford. "Postural and respiratory functions of the pelvic floor muscles." Neurourology and Urodynamics 26 (2007): 362-371.

10. Junginger B., K. Baessler, and R. Sapsford. "Effect of abdominal and pelvic floor tasks on muscle activity, abdominal pressure and bladder neck." International Urogynecology Journal 21 (2010): 69-77.

11. Balogh, A. "Pilates and pregnancy." Midwives 8, no. 5 (2007): 220-222.

12. Memon, H. U., and V. L. Handa. "Vaginal childbirth and pelvic floor disorders." Women's Health 9, no. 3 (2013): 265-277.

13. Deering, S. A Practical Manual to Labor and Delivery for Medical Students and Residents. Xlibris Corporation, 2009.

14. Bewyer, K. J., D. C. Bewyer, and D. Messenger. "Pilot data: association between gluteus medius weakness and low back pain during pregnancy." The Iowa Orthopaedic Journal 29 (2009): 97-99.

15. Hart, M. A. "Help! My orthopaedic patient is pregnant!" Orthopaedic Nursing 24, no. 2 (2005): 108-116.

16. Benjamin, D. R., A. T. M. van de Water, and C. L. Peiris. "Effects of exercise on diastasis of the rectus abdominis muscle in the antenatal and postnatal periods: a systematic review." Physiotherapy 100, no. 1 (2014): 1-8.

17. Kawaguchi, J. K., and R. K. Pickering. "Population-Specific Concerns-The Pregnant Athlete, Part 1: Anatomy and Physiology of Pregnancy." Athletic Therapy Today 15, no. 2 (2010): 39-43.

18. Foti, T., J. R. Davids, and A. Bagley. "A Biomechanical Analysis of Gait During Pregnancy." The Journal of Bone & Joint Surgery 82, no. 5 (2000): 625-632.

19. Zachovajevas, P., B. Zachovajevienė, and J. Banionytė. "Physical therapy and maternity support garment: influence on core stability and low back pain during pregnancy and after delivery." Education Physical Activity Sport 86 (2012): 99-106.

20. Abduljalil, K., P. Furness, T. N, Johnson, A. Rostami-Hodjegan, and H. Soltani. "Anatomical, Physiological and Metabolic Changeswith Gestational Age during Normal Pregnancy." Clinical Pharmacokinetics 51, no. 6 (2012): 365-396.

21. Melzer, K., Y. Schutz, M. Boulvain, and B. Kayser. "Physical Activity and Pregnancy." Sports Medicine 40, no. 6 (2010): 493-507.

22. Oatridge, A., A. Holdcroft, and N. Saeed. "Change in brain size during and after pregnancy: study in healthy women and women with preeclampsia." American Journal of Neuroradiology 23 (2002): 19-26.

23. Sneag, D. B., and J. A. Bendo. "Pregnancy-related Low Back Pain." Orthopedics 30, no. 10 (2007): 839-847.

24. Armitage, N. H., and D. A. Smart. "Changes in Air Force Fitness Measurements Pre- and Post-Childbirth." Military Medicine 177, no. 12 (2012): 1519-1523.

25. Hodges, P.W., J. E. Butler, and D. K. McKenzie. "Contraction of the human diaphragm during rapid postural adjustments." The Journal of Physiology 505, no. 2 (1997): 539-548.

26. Madill, S. "Differences in pelvic floor muscle activation and functional output between women with and without stress urinary incontinence." Thesis, Queen's University, 2009. http://qspace.library.queensu.ca/dspace/handle/1974/5185.

27. Hodges, P.W., and C. A. Richardson. "Feedforward contraction of transversus abdominis is not influenced by the direction of arm movement." Experimental Brain Research 114, no. 2 (1997): 362-370.

28. Sapsford, R. R., and P. W. Hodges. "The effect of abdominal and pelvic floor muscle activation on urine flow in women." International Urogynecology Journal 23, no. 9 (2012): 1225-1230.

29. Pereira, L. C., S. Botelho, and J. Marques. "Are transversus abdominis/oblique internal and pelvic floor muscles coactivated during pregnancy and postpartum?" Neurourology and Urodynamics 32, no. 5 (2013): 416-419.

30. Kim, E. Y., S. Y. Kim, and D. W. Oh. "Pelvic floor muscle exercises utilizing trunk stabilization for treating postpartum urinary incontinence: randomized controlled pilot trial of supervised versus unsupervised training." Clinical Rehabilitation 26, no. 2 (2012): 132-141.

31. Kawaguchi, J. K., and R. K. Pickering. "The Pregnant Athlete, Part 3: Exercise in the Postpartum Period and Return to Play." Athletic Therapy Today 15, no. (2010): 36-41.

32. Hodges, P. "Transversus abdominis: a different view of the elephant." British Journal of Sports Medicine 42, no. 12 (2008): 941-944.

33. Neumann, P., and V. Gill. "Pelvic floor and abdominal muscle interaction: EMG activity and intra-abdominal pressure." International Urogynecology Journal 13 (2002): 125-132.

34. Larson-Meyer, E. "The effects of regular postpartum exercise on mother and child: review article." International SportMed Journal 4, no. 6 (2003): 1-14.

35. Gaston, A., and K. L. Gammage. "Health versus appearance messages, self-monitoring and pregnant women's intentions to exercise postpartum." Journal of Reproductive and Infant Psychology 28, no. 4 (2010): 345-358.

36. Evenson, K. R., A. H. Herring, and F. Wen. "Self-reported and objectively measured physical activity among a cohort of postpartum women: the PIN postpartum study." Journal of Physical Activity & Health 9 (2012): 5-20.

37. Lovelady, C. A, M. J. Bopp, H. L. Colleran, H. K. Mackie, an L. Wideman. "Effect of Exercise Training on Loss of Bone Mineral Density during Lactation." Medicine & Science in Sports & Exercise 41, no. 10 (2009): 1902-1907.

38. Fryar, C. D., M. D. Carroll, and C. L. Ogden. "Prevalence of overweight, obesity, and extreme obesity among adults: United States, trends 1960–1962 through 2009–2010." National Center for Health Statistics, Health-E Stats (2012). http://www.cdc.gov/nchs/data/hestat/obesity_adult_09_10/obesity_adult_09_10.htm.

39. Meyer, D. L. "Effect of Postpartum Exercise on Mothers and their Offspring: A Review of the Literature." Obesity Research 10, no. 8 (2002): 841-853.

40. Lovelady, C. "Balancing exercise and food intake with lactation to promote post-partum weight loss." Proceedings of the Nutrition Society 70, no. 2 (2011): 181-184.

41. Adegboye, A. A., and Y. M. Linne. "Diet or exercise, or both, for weight reduction in women after childbirth." Cochrane Dadatase of Systematic Reviews 7 (2013): 1-67.

42. Berne, Robert M, and Matthew N Levy. Principles of Physiology, Mosby, 2000.

43. Mayberry, L. J., J. A. Horowitz, and E. Declercq. "Depression Symptom Prevalence and Demographic Risk Factors Among U.S. Women During the First 2 Years Postpartum." Journal of Obstetric, Gynecologic, & Neonatal Nursing 36, no. 6 (2007): 542-549.

44. Gavin, N. I., B. N. Gaynes, and K. N. Lohr. "Perinatal depression: a systematic review of prevalence and incidence." Obstetrics & Gynecology 106, no. 5 (2005): 1071-1083.

45. Norman, E., M. Sherburn, and R. H. Osborne. "An Exercise and Education Program Improves Well-Being of New Mothers: A Randomized Controlled Trial." Physical Therapy 90, no. 3 (2010): 348-355.

46. Haruna, M. "The effects of an exercise program on health-related quality of life in postpartum mothers: A randomized controlled trial." Health 5, no. 3 (2013): 432-439.

47. Ko, Y. L., C. L. Yang, C. L. Fang, M. Y. Lee, and P. C. Lin. "Community-based postpartum exercise program." Journal of Clinical Nursing 22 No. 15-16 (2013): 2122-2131.

48. Dritsa, M., D. Costa, G. Dupuis, I. Lowensteyn, and S. Khalifé. "Effects of a Home-based Exercise Intervention on Fatigue in Postpartum Depressed Women: Results of a Randomized Controlled Trial." Annals of Behavioral Medicine 35, no. 2 (2008): 179-187.

49. Mokdad, A. H., J. S. Marks, D. F. Stroup, and J. L. Gerberding. "Actual Causes of Death in the United States, 2000." The Journal of the American Medical Association 291, no. 10 (2004): 1238-1245.

50. Centers For Disease Control and Prevention. "Obesity Facts." Adolescent and School Health, last modified April 24, 2015. http://www.cdc.gov/healthyyouth/obesity/facts.htm.

51. Whitaker, R. C., J. A. Wright, M. S. Pepe, K. D. Seidel, and W. H. Dietz. "Predicting obesity in young adulthood from childhood and parental obesity." New England Journal of Medicine 337, no. 13 (1997): 869-873.

52. Østbye, T., K. M. Krause, M. Stroo, et al. "Parent-focused change to prevent obesity in preschoolers: Results from the KAN-DO study." Preventive Medicine 55, no. 3 (2012): 188-195.

53. Craig, C. L., C. Cameron, and C. Tudor-Locke. "Relationship between parent and child pedometer-determined physical activity: a sub-study of the CANPLAY surveillance study." International Journal of Behavioral Nutrition and Physical Activity 10, no. 8 (2013): 1-8.

54. Jacobi, D., A. Caille, J. M. Borys, et al. "Parent-Offspring Correlations in Pedometer-Assessed Physical Activity." PLOS ONE 6, no. 12 (2011).

55. Oliver, M., G. M. Schofield, and P. J. Schluter. "Parent influences on preschoolers' objectively assessed physical activity." Journal of Science and Medicine in Sport 13, no. 4 (2010): 403-409.

56. Campbell, K. J., and K. D. Hesketh. "Strategies which aim to positively impact on weight, physical activity, diet and sedentary behaviours in children from zero to five years. A systematic review of the literature." Obesity Reviews 8, no. 4 (2007): 327-338.

57. Malina, R. M. "Tracking of physical activity and physical fitness across the lifespan." Research Quarterly for Exercise and Sport 67, no. S3 (1996): 48-57.

58. Hesketh, K. R., L. Goodfellow, U. Ekelund, et al. "Activity Levels in Mothers and Their Preschool Children." PEDIATRICS 133, no. 4 (2014): e973-e980.

59. Fuemmeler, B. F., C. B. Anderson, and L. C. Mâsse. "Parent-child relationship of directly measured physical activity." International Journal of Behavioral Nutrition and Physical Activity 8, no. 1 (2011): 17.

60. Jago, R., K. R. Fox, A. S. Page, R. Brockman, and J. L. Thompson. "Parent and child physical activity and sedentary time: Do active parents foster active children?" BMC Public Health 10, no. 1 (2010): 194.

61. Braithwaite, I., A. W. Stewart, R. J. Hancox, and R. Beasley. "The worldwide association between television viewing and obesity in children and adolescents: cross sectional study." PLOS ONE 8, no. 9 (2013).

62. Oliver, M., G. M. Schofield, and P. J. Schluter. "Parent influences on preschoolers' objectively assessed physical activity." Journal of Science and Medicine in Sport 13 (2010): 403-409.

63. Kalakanis, L. E., G. S. Goldfield, R. A. Paluch, and L. H. Epstein. "Parental activity as a determinant of activity level and patterns of activity in obese children." Research Quarterly for Exercise and Sport 72, no. 3 (2001): 202-209.

64. Rosenkranz, R. R. "Maternal physical-activity-related parenting behaviors may influence children's physical activity levels and relative weight." Women in Sport and Physical Activity Journal 20, no. 1 (2011): 3-12.

65. Tucker, P., M. M van Zandvoort, S. M. Burke, and J. D. Irwin. "The influence of parents and the home environment on preschoolers 'physical activity behaviours: A qualitative investigation of childcare providers' perspectives." BMC Public Health 11, no. 1 (2011): 168.

66. Lovelady, C. A., K. E. Garner, and K. L. Moreno. "The effect of weight loss in overweight, lactating women on the growth of their infants." New England Journal of Medicine 342, no. 7 (2000): 449-453.

67. Dewey, K. G. "Effects of maternal caloric restriction and exercise during lactation." The Journal of Nutrition 128, no. 2S (1998): S386.

68. Lederman, S.A. "Influence of lactation on body weight regulation." Nutrition reviews 62, no. 7 (2004): S112-S119.

69. Dewey, K. G., and C. A. Lovelady. "A randomized study of the effects of aerobic exercise by lactating women on breast-milk volume and composition." New England Journal of Medicine 330, no. 7 (1994): 449-453.

70. Adair, L. S., and B. M. Popkin. "Prolonged lactation contributes to depletion of maternal energy reserves in Filipino women." The Journal of Nutrition 122, no. 8 (1992): 1643-1655.

71. Panter-Brick, C. "Seasonality of energy expenditure during pregnancy and lactation for rural Nepali women." The American Journal of Clinical Nutrition 57 (1993): 620-628.

72. Sanders, M. J., and T. Morse. "The Ergonomics of Caring for Children: An Exploratory Study." American Journal of Occupational Therapy 59, no. 3 (2005): 285-295.

73. Skaggs, C. D., H. Prather, G. Gross, J. W. George, P. A. Thompson, and D. M. Nelson. "Back and Pelvic Pain in an Underserved United States Pregnant Population: A Preliminary Descriptive Survey." Journal of Manipulative and Physiological Therapeutics 30, no. 2 (2007): 130-134.

74. Stuber, K., S. Wynd, and C. A. Weis. "Adverse events from spinal manipulation in the pregnant and postpartum periods: a critical review of the literature." Chiropractic & Manual Therapies 20, no. 1 (2012): 8-16.

75. Thein-Nissenbaum, J. M., E. F. Thompson, E. S. Chumanov, and B. Heiderscheit. "Low Back and Hip Pain in a Postpartum Runner: Applying Ultrasound Imaging and Running Analysis." Journal of Orthopaedic & Sports Physical Therapy 42, no. 7 (2012): 615-624.

76. Fritz, J. M., J. A. Cleland, and J. D. Childs. "Subgrouping Patients With Low Back Pain: Evolution of a Classification Approach to Physical Therapy." Journal of Orthopaedic & Sports Physical Therapy 37, no. 6 (2007): 290-302.

77. Jensen, M. C., and M. N. Brant-Zawadzki. "Magnetic resonance imaging of the lumbar spine in people without back pain." New England Journal of Medicine 331, no. 2 (1994): 69-73.

78. Delitto, A., R. E. Erhard, and R. W. Bowling. "A Treatment-Based Classification Approach to Low Back Syndrome: Identifying and Staging Patients for Conservative Treatment." Physical Therapy 75, no. 6 (1995): 470-485.

79. Henry, S. M., J. M. Fritz, A. R. Trombley, and J. Y. Bunn. "Reliability of a Treatment-Based Classification System for Subgrouping People With Low Back Pain." Journal of Orthopaedic & Sports Physical Therapy 42, no. 9 (2012): 797-805.

80. Fritz, J. M., A. Delitto, and R. E. Erhard. "Comparison of Classification-Based Physical Therapy With Therapy Based on Clinical Practice Guidelines for Patients with Acute Low Back Pain: A Randomized Clinical Trial." Spine 28, no. 13 (2003): 1363.

81. Sato, K., and M. Mokha." Does Core Strength Training Influence Running Kinetics, Lower Extremity Stability, and 5000m Performance in Runners?" The Journal of Strength & Conditioning Research 23, no. 1 (2009): 133-140.

82. Rajalakshmi, D., and N. S. Kumar. "Strengthening Transversus Abdominis in Pregnancy Related Pelvic Pain: The Pressure Biofeedback Stabilization Training." Global Journal of Health Science 4, no. 4 (2012).

83. Kanakaris, N. K., C. S. Roberts, and P. V. Giannoudis. "Pregnancy-related pelvic girdle pain: an update." BMC Medicine 9, no. 1 (2011): 15.

84. Weibe, J. "The Diaphragm-Pelvic Floor Piston for Rehab and Fitness Professionals." Julie Wiebe PT, last modified June 16, 2014. https://www.juliewiebept.com/store-video/the-diaphragm-pelvic-floor-piston-for-rehab-and-fitness-protected/.

85. Sahakian, J., and S. Woodward. "Stress incontinence and pelvic floor exercises in pregnancy." British Journal of Nursing 21, no. 18 (2012): S10-S15.

86. Shelly, B. "Introduction to Rehabilitation of Pelvic Floor Dysfunction and Urinary Incontinence." Continuing Education Course, Allied Health Education Online Training, August 11, 2014.

87. Romano, M., A. Cacciatore, and R. Giordano. "Postpartum period: three distinct but continuous phases." Journal of Prenatal Medicine 4, no. 2 (2010): 22-25.

88. Whitehouse, T. "Managing stress incontinence in postnatal women." Nursing Time 108, no. 18-19 (2012): 16-18.

89. Opala-Berdzik, A., and S. Dąbrowski. "Physiotherapy in diastasis of the rectus muscles of abdomen in women during pregnancy and postpartum." Physiotherapy 17, no. 4 (2009).

90. Mesquita, L. A., A. V. Machado, and A. V. Andrade. "Fisioterapia para redução da diástase dos músculos retos abdominais no pós-parto." The Revista Brasileira de Ginecologia e Obstetrícia 21, no. 5 (1999): 267-272.

91. Riddle, D.L., M. Pulisic, P. Pidcoe, and R.E. Johnson. "Risk factors for plantar fasciitis: a matched case-control study." The Journal of Bone & Joint Surgery 85, no. 5 (2003): 872-877.

92. Uden, H., E. Boesch, and S. Kumar. "Plantar fasciitis—to jab or to support? A systematic review of the current best evidence." Journal of Multidisciplinary Healthcare 4 (2011): 155-1164.

93. Hyland, M.R., A. Webber-Gaffney, L. Cohen, and S. W. Lichtman. "Randomized Controlled Trial of Calcaneal Taping, Sham Taping, and Plantar Fascia Stretching for the Short-Term Management of Plantar Heel Pain." Journal of Orthopaedic & Sports Physical Therapy 36, no. 6 (2006): 364-371.

94. Gerritsen, A., M. de Krom, M. A. Struijs, R. Scholten, H. de Vet, and L. M. Bouter. "Conservative treatment options for carpal tunnel syndrome: a systematic review of randomised controlled trials." Journal of Neurology 249, no. 3 (2002): 272-280.

95. Kim, P., H. Lee, T. Kim, and I. Jeon. "Current Approaches for Carpal Tunnel Syndrome." Clinics in Orthopedic Surgery 6, no. 3 (2014): 253.

96. Zyluk, A. "Carpal tunnel syndrome in pregnancy: A review." Polish Orthopedics & Traumatology 78 (2012): 223-227.

97. Zyluk, A. "Is carpal tunnel syndrome an occupational disease? A review." Polish Orthopedics & Traumatology 78 (2012): 121-126.

98. Petit Le Manac'h, A., Y. Roquelaure, C. Ha, et al. "Risk factors for de Quervain's disease in a French working population". Scandinavian Journal of Work, Environment & Health 37, no. 5 (2011): 394-401.

99. Anderson, S. E., and L. S. Steinbach. "'Baby wrist': MRI of an overuse syndrome in mothers." American Journal of Roentgenology 182, no. 3 (2004): 719-724.

100. McGuire, D K, B D Levine, J W Williamson, P G Snell, C Gunnar Blomqvist, B Saltin, and J H Mitchell. "A 30-Year Follow-Up of the Dallas Bed Rest and Training Study II. Effect of Age on Cardiovascular Adaptation to Exercise Training." Circulation 104, no. 12 (September 18, 2001): 1358–66.

Made in the USA
Middletown, DE
24 February 2020